OTHER BOOKS BY
DRS. RACHAEL AND RICHARD HELLER

The *Carbohydrate Addict's Calorie Counter*
The *Carbohydrate Addict's Carbohydrate Counter*

The *Carbohydrate Addict's Diet*
The *Carbohydrate Addict's Gram Counter*
Carbohydrate-Addicted Kids
The *Carbohydrate Addict's LifeSpan Program*
The *Carbohydrate Addict's Healthy for Life Plan*
The *Carbohydrate Addict's Healthy Heart Program*
The *Carbohydrate Addict's Program for Success*

Visit the Hellers at their website at:
www.carbohydrateaddicts.com

THE CARBOHYDRATE ADDICT'S FAT COUNTER

DR. RACHAEL F. HELLER
ASSISTANT PROFESSOR EMERITUS, MT. SINAI SCHOOL OF MEDICINE·
ASSISTANT PROFESSOR EMERITUS, GRADUATE CENTER OF THE
CITY UNIVERSITY OF NEW YORK

DR. RICHARD F. HELLER
PROFESSOR EMERITUS, MT. SINAI SCHOOL OF MEDICINE·
PROFESSOR EMERITUS, GRADUATE CENTER OF THE
CITY UNIVERSITY OF NEW YORK·
PROFESSOR EMERITUS, CITY UNIVERSITY OF NEW YORK

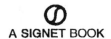

A SIGNET BOOK

A Note to the Reader
The ideas and data contained in this book are not intended as a substitute for
medical treatment by a physician The reader should regularly consult a physician
in matters relating to health

SIGNET
Published by New American Library, a division of
Penguin Putnam Inc , 375 Hudson Street,
New York, New York 10014, U S A.
Penguin Books Ltd, 27 Wrights Lane, London W8 5TZ, England
Penguin Books Australia Ltd, Ringwood, Victoria, Australia
Penguin Books Canada Ltd, 10 Alcorn Avenue, Toronto, Ontario, Canada M4V 3B2
Penguin Books (N Z) Ltd, 182–190 Wairau Road, Auckland 10, New Zealand

Penguin Books Ltd, Registered Offices
Harmondsworth, Middlesex, England

First published by Signet, an imprint of New American Library,
a division of Penguin Putnam Inc.

First Printing, January 2000
10 9 8 7 6 5 4 3 2 1

**You are about to discover a
FAT COUNTER
like none you have ever seen!**

The 4000 food comparisons* in this counter are presented in two new and exciting reader-friendly formats

Gone are the endless rows of tiny numbers that require the use of higher math and calculators before you can make a food choice.

A revolution in counters, these simple designs present food counts in clear, easy-to-read graphs that will make you exclaim, "Wow! Now I can see it all—at a glance!"

A-to-Z charts, found in the front of this counter, list foods in alphabetical order within several major categories. This format will help you to quickly and easily find a particular food by its name. Numbers at the end of each bar indicate specific grams of fat.

Hi-Low Comparison charts, found in the second half of this counter, rank foods from low to high. This format will help you to effortlessly select a "best choice" from any given category of foods. Again, numbers at the end of each bar indicate the specific grams of fat.

All the Carbohydrate Addict's Counters give you the information you need to put you in control and to make gram and calorie counting exciting and fun!

*Nutritional values in this counter were taken from material supplied by or direct communication with the US Department of Agriculture, scientific studies, computer data banks, and representatives of the food industry When counts, as provided by a variety of sources, differ one from the other, an average or typical count is calculated and used All data are rounded to the nearest whole number Neither the authors nor publisher assume any responsibility for any errors contained herein and all readers must work in accordance with and in conjunction with their own personal physician For information on abbreviations, see the introductory pages that follow

CONTENTS

INTRODUCTION

Are You Addicted to Carbohydrates?

After breakfast, are you hungry before it's time for lunch? Once you start to eat breads and other starches, snack foods or sweets, do you have a very difficult time stopping? Do you snack when you're not really hungry? If so, it is likely that you are a carbohydrate addict. You may respond differently to that bread or pasta or potato, to those snack foods or sweets, than other people do.

Researchers have begun to confirm what many of us knew all along, that when it comes to eating and weight, as in so many other things, each of us is different. C. Everett Koop, M.D., the former Surgeon General of the United States, notes that some of us are "carbohydrate sensitive." As many as 75 percent of the overweight, and a good percentage of normal-weight individuals as well, appear to have a physical imbalance that leads to an addiction to carbohydrates.

Carbohydrate addiction is the result of an imbalance in the hormone insulin, and this "hunger hormone" makes us crave carbohydrate-rich foods intensely and repeatedly.

If you are addicted to carbohydrates, it is not your fault! Those of us who are carbohydrate addicts have genes that make us exceptionally good at storing carbohydrates in the form of fat. No matter how great our desire to stop eating and lose weight, our bodies seem to fight us at every level. Our basic constitution makes carbohydrate-rich foods taste exceptionally good and makes us more likely to put on weight and keep it on.

If you are addicted to carbohydrates, we hope you come to understand that carbohydrate addiction is not a matter of will-power but of biology. Your cravings and weight gain are symptoms of an underlying physical imbalance. We know what causes it and now we know how to correct it.

Carbohydrate addicts often find that:

- Once they start to eat bread, pasta, or other starches, snack foods or sweets, they have a difficult time stopping.
- After a full breakfast, they get hungry before lunch.
- They get tired and/or hungry in the mid-afternoon and a snack makes them feel better.
- They gain weight easily and/or, after dieting, tend to quickly gain weight back.
- They continue to eat or snack when they are not hungry.
- They sometimes lose control of their eating.

If, like so many others, you are addicted to carbohydrates, it is no mystery to us why you have struggled to stay on diet after diet, why diets often fail to help you keep the weight off, and why you may suffer from insulin-related health problems.

If you are a carbohydrate addict, starches, snack foods, junk foods and sweets may hold the key to your addiction and to your victory as well. On our Programs, you will find that you can enjoy these foods every day, in satisfying quantities.

For our Programs' essential guidelines, see *The Carbohydrate Addict's LifeSpan Program* (Plume), *The Carbohydrate Addict's Healthy for Life Plan* (Plume), *The Carbohydrate Addict's Diet* (Signet) or *The Carbohydrate Addict's Healthy Heart Program* (Ballantine). Our companion workbook, *The Carbohydrate Addict's Program for Success* (Plume), offers help with the emotional and spiritual aspects of carbohydrate addiction, and our other Carbohydrate Addict's Counters (Signet) can provide vital facts for success.

A Special Message from the Authors

Both of us were overweight children and adolescents. In time, as predicted, we became overweight adults. We grew up knowing the caloric content of foods as well as we knew the multiplication tables. And each of us, independently, struggled with calorie counters for as long as we can remember.

The calorie counters of three decades ago were uninteresting little books filled with columns of tiny numbers that were confusing to look at, difficult to read, and impossible to remember. After a tedious search for a food value, we easily forgot it by the next day. Comparing the calorie content of one food to another seemed to require the intelligence of a rocket scientist.

How could anyone be expected to compare ⅓ cup of one cereal with one ounce of another cereal? In some cases, milk and sugar were included, in other cases they were not.

As authors ourselves, we now understand that the writers who compiled these books included noncomparable quantities because doing so was a quick and easy way to take information directly from databases. In the past as now, we think this short-cutting does a terrible disservice to the reader.

Surprisingly, most of today's calorie counters do not look much different, nor are they any easier to use, than those counters of three decades ago. Many people have come to expect that calorie counting is a tedious necessity employed in the attainment of one's health and weight-loss goals.

We have found the opposite to be true and we think that you will too!

You are about to discover that calorie counting—and comparing—can be fun. In the Carbohydrate Addict's Counters, comparisons of calories, carbohydrates, and fats, respectively, become meaningful and easily understood.

In an instant you will be able to visualize the caloric contents of the entire aisle of cereals on your supermarket shelves. You will be able to intelligently choose the best meat for your weight-loss or health-related goals, and you will be able to select, with confidence, the dessert that is "worth" the calories. Fast food restaurants will now present a range of offerings, some of which will prove to be surprisingly better choices. The nutritional and caloric contents of meats, vegetables, snacks, sweets, and thousands of other foods become easy to grasp and hold in your mind.

Best of all, you will grow more confident with each success you achieve.

Between the two of us, we have lost over two hundred pounds, and we have maintained our ideal weights for over fifteen years. We are in perfect health for the first time in our lives, and our energy is unbounded.

We wish for you the permanent weight-loss and ideal health that we have achieved after so many years of struggle. The challenges of the past have made our present success that much sweeter.

What Is Dietary Fat?

Fat is one of the body's necessary nutrients (the others being carbohydrates and proteins). All forms of fat are made up of a combination of building blocks called fatty acids. These building blocks can remain unattached as single molecules (free fatty acids) or may be assembled into groupings that form larger molecules (fats). A saturated fat is a fat in which each molecule is filled to capacity with hydrogen. When there is one opening for an atom in each molecule, the fat is said to be monounsaturated. When there are several openings for hydrogen in each molecule, the fat is said to be polyunsaturated.

In general, saturated fats come from animal sources and remain solid at room temperature. Some tropical oils, such as coconut oil and palm oil, are exceptions to the solid-saturated-fat rule. These two saturated oils are semi-solid at room temperature and come from plant sources.

A diet high in saturated fats has been shown to increase the risk of heart disease and some forms of cancer. It is important to remember that it is not advisable to make any changes in your dietary choices without first discussing this matter with your physician.

How Much Fat Should I Eat?

The American Heart Association, in its Eating Plan for Healthy Americans, offers the following nutritional guidelines:

- Total fat intake should be no more than 30 percent of total calories.

- Saturated fatty acid intake should be 8–10 percent of total calories.
- Polyunsaturated fatty acid intake should be up to 10 percent of total calories.
- Monounsaturated fatty acids should make up to 15 percent of total calories.
- Cholesterol intake should be less than 300 milligrams per day.

As always, individual needs must be considered, so check with your physician before making any dietary or lifestyle changes.

For purposes of calculation, each gram of fat contains 9 calories.

How Much Should I Weigh? Three Tests to See If You're Overweight

Your height, age, muscle mass, and weight distribution all influence your weight and help determine the best weight for you. Physicians and researchers generally recommend three ways of determining your ideal weight.

Test #1: Weight Range Charts

The first way to determine your ideal weight is by consulting a published chart of desirable weights. The standardized chart on the following page is used by the United States Department of Agriculture.

Test #2: Pinch an Inch

While weight-range charts can help you to determine whether you have a weight problem, they cannot tell the whole story. Some people weigh more than the chart indicates to be "desirable," but their excess weight is primarily attributable to muscle mass. Others may find that they are not overweight according to the chart but are concerned that the placement of those extra pounds puts them in the "need to lose" category.

If you want to try a simple and quick test, pinch a fold of

RANGE OF "DESIRABLE" WEIGHTS*

Height without shoes	Weight without clothes	
	Men (pounds)	Women (pounds)
4'10"		92–121
4'11"		95–124
5'0"		98–127
5'1"	105–134	101–130
5'2"	108–137	104–134
5'3"	111–141	107–138
5'4"	114–145	110–142
5'5"	117–149	114–146
5'6"	121–154	118–150
5'7"	125–159	122–154
5'8"	129–163	126–159
5'9"	133–167	130–164
5'10"	137–172	134–169
5'11"	141–177	
6'0"	145–182	
6'1"	149–187	
6'2"	153–192	
6'3"	157–197	

*United States Department of Agriculture Human Nutrition Information Service Agriculture, Information Bulletin 364

skin at the back of your upper arm. If you can pinch more than an inch, you are probably carrying more weight (in the form of fat) than is desirable.

Test #3: Body Mass Index (BMI)
Most scientists and physicians have started to use Body Mass Index Scores as a way to get a better picture of an individual's weight level. Designed as a tool for statistical analysis, the BMI can help health professionals make evaluations regarding health risk factors related to excess weight.

Using a mathematical formula, the BMI takes into account both a person's weight and height. BMI equals a person's weight in kilograms divided by height in meters squared (BMI=kg/m^2). But don't worry, the table that follows will make it easy for you to get your BMI score.

To use the BMI table that follows, find your height (in inches) in the left-hand column. Move across the row to your weight. The number at the bottom of your weight column is your Body Mass Index (BMI).

BODY MASS INDEX CHART

Height (in.)

58	91	96	100	105	110	115	119	124	129	134	138	143	167	191
59	94	99	104	109	114	119	124	128	133	138	143	148	173	198
60	97	102	107	112	118	123	128	133	138	143	148	153	179	204
61	100	106	111	116	122	127	132	137	143	148	153	158	185	211
62	104	109	115	120	126	131	136	142	147	153	158	164	191	218
63	107	113	118	124	130	135	141	146	152	158	163	169	197	225
64	110	116	122	128	134	140	145	151	157	163	169	174	204	232
65	114	120	126	132	138	144	150	156	162	168	174	180	210	240
66	118	124	130	136	142	148	155	161	167	173	179	186	216	247
67	121	127	134	140	146	153	159	166	172	178	185	191	223	255
68	125	131	138	144	151	158	164	171	177	184	190	197	230	262
69	138	135	142	149	155	162	169	176	182	189	196	203	236	270
70	132	139	146	153	160	167	174	181	188	195	202	207	243	278
71	136	143	150	157	165	172	179	186	193	200	208	215	250	286
72	140	147	154	162	169	177	184	191	199	206	213	221	258	294
73	144	151	159	166	174	182	189	197	204	212	219	227	265	302
74	148	155	163	171	179	186	194	202	210	218	225	233	272	311
75	152	160	168	176	184	192	200	208	216	224	232	240	279	319
76	156	164	172	180	189	197	205	213	221	230	238	246	287	328
BMI (kg/m^2)	19	20	21	22	23	24	25	26	27	28	29	30	35	40

Using your BMI score, the chart below can help you to better determine your weight level.

BMI (Body Mass Index)	Weight Assessment
18.5 or less	Underweight
18.5–24.9	Normal
25.0–29.9	Overweight
30.0–39.9	Obese
40 or greater	Extremely Obese

What This Book Can Do For You

All of the Carbohydrate Addict's Counters provide a whole new way of looking at food values—a simple and fun way to keep track of your eating and help you to make healthful choices.

We hope that this counter will become a good and well-used friend. It carries with it the experiences of over half a million people, along with our best wishes for a long, healthy, and happy life.

An Important Note

Any change in diet should be made in consultation with your physician. The data contained herein are not intended to replace medical advice. Any questions or concerns should be addressed to your physician.

What Really Counts

Of all the important tools that are available to you, the most important by far is the commitment you bring to making your dreams come true.

So choose the best foods for you, plan and prepare healthful meals and, as appropriate, keep count of the fats you consume. In the counting, make certain to count on yourself—your strength, your love of life, and your desire to make your body and your life happy and healthy You are your most important resource.

ABBREVIATIONS YOU'LL FIND IN
THE CARBOHYDRATE ADDICT'S COUNTERS

When You See This Abbreviation. . . .	It Means This
/	or
bl cheese	blue cheese
broc	broccoli
ch	cheese
dress	dressing
env	envelope
fl	fluid or flavor
flav	flavor(s)
Fr dress	French dressing
frzn	frozen
G'ma's Big	Grandma's Big
marg	margarine
parm	parmesan
Pepperidge	Pepperidge Farm
pkg	package
pkt	packet
q'tr pnd'r	quarter pounder
reg	regular
saus	sausage
Stella D	Stella D'Oro
sweet'd	sweetened
Thous Island	Thousand Island
tom	tomato
veg	vegetable
w/	with
wh	white

THE
CARBOHYDRATE
ADDICT'S
FAT
COUNTER

ALPHABETICAL CHARTS

BEVERAGES*, Part 1

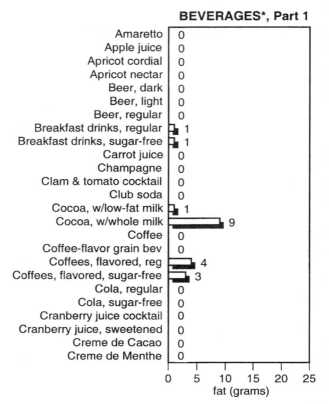

	fat (grams)
Amaretto	0
Apple juice	0
Apricot cordial	0
Apricot nectar	0
Beer, dark	0
Beer, light	0
Beer, regular	0
Breakfast drinks, regular	1
Breakfast drinks, sugar-free	1
Carrot juice	0
Champagne	0
Clam & tomato cocktail	0
Club soda	0
Cocoa, w/low-fat milk	1
Cocoa, w/whole milk	9
Coffee	0
Coffee-flavor grain bev	0
Coffees, flavored, reg	4
Coffees, flavored, sugar-free	3
Cola, regular	0
Cola, sugar-free	0
Cranberry juice cocktail	0
Cranberry juice, sweetened	0
Creme de Cacao	0
Creme de Menthe	0

* Counts for non-alcoholic drinks and beer are based on
8-fluid-ounce servings, for wine on 3 1/2-fluid-ounce
servings and, for hard liquor, on 1 1/2-fluid-ounce servings.

2

BEVERAGES*, Part 2

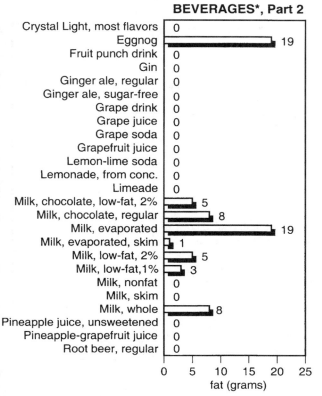

	fat (grams)
Crystal Light, most flavors	0
Eggnog	19
Fruit punch drink	0
Gin	0
Ginger ale, regular	0
Ginger ale, sugar-free	0
Grape drink	0
Grape juice	0
Grape soda	0
Grapefruit juice	0
Lemon-lime soda	0
Lemonade, from conc.	0
Limeade	0
Milk, chocolate, low-fat, 2%	5
Milk, chocolate, regular	8
Milk, evaporated	19
Milk, evaporated, skim	1
Milk, low-fat, 2%	5
Milk, low-fat,1%	3
Milk, nonfat	0
Milk, skim	0
Milk, whole	8
Pineapple juice, unsweetened	0
Pineapple-grapefruit juice	0
Root beer, regular	0

* Counts for non-alcoholic drinks and beer are based on
8-fluid-ounce servings, for wine on 3 1/2-fluid-ounce
servings and, for hard liquor, on 1 1/2-fluid-ounce servings.

BEVERAGES*, Part 3

Beverage	fat (grams)
Root beer, sugar-free	0
Rum	0
7 Up, regular	0
7 Up, sugar-free	0
Shake, chocolate, thick	6
Shake, vanilla, thick	7
Slim Fast, most flav, 11 fl oz	3
Soy milk	5
Sprite, regular	0
Sprite, sugar-free	0
Tea	0
Tomato juice, 8 fl oz	0
Tonic water, regular	0
Tonic water, sugar-free	0
Vegetable juice cocktail	0
Vegetable juice, V-8	0
Vodka	0
Whisky	0
Wine, dessert	0
Wine, port	0
Wine, red	0
Wine, sherry	0
Wine, white	0
Yoo-Hoo, chocolate drink	1

fat (grams) 0 5 10 15 20 25

* Counts for non-alcoholic drinks and beer are based on
8-fluid-ounce servings, for wine on 3 1/2-fluid-ounce
servings and, for hard liquor, on 1 1/2-fluid-ounce servings.

**Bread, Crackers, and Flours:
BAGELS***

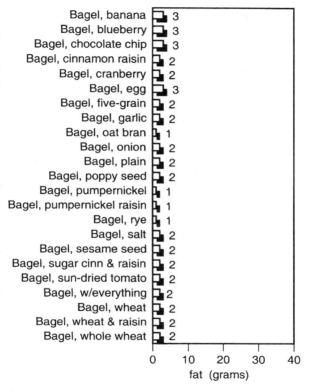

Bagel, banana	3
Bagel, blueberry	3
Bagel, chocolate chip	3
Bagel, cinnamon raisin	2
Bagel, cranberry	2
Bagel, egg	3
Bagel, five-grain	2
Bagel, garlic	2
Bagel, oat bran	1
Bagel, onion	2
Bagel, plain	2
Bagel, poppy seed	2
Bagel, pumpernickel	1
Bagel, pumpernickel raisin	1
Bagel, rye	1
Bagel, salt	2
Bagel, sesame seed	2
Bagel, sugar cinn & raisin	2
Bagel, sun-dried tomato	2
Bagel, w/everything	2
Bagel, wheat	2
Bagel, wheat & raisin	2
Bagel, whole wheat	2

0   10   20   30   40

fat (grams)

* Counts are based on one bagel, approximate weight:
3 ounces.

Bread, Crackers, and Flours:
BISCUITS, ROLLS & MUFFINS*

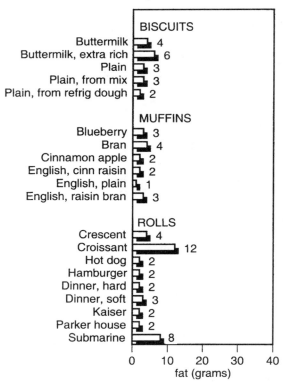

BISCUITS

	fat (grams)
Buttermilk	4
Buttermilk, extra rich	6
Plain	3
Plain, from mix	3
Plain, from refrig dough	2

MUFFINS

	fat (grams)
Blueberry	3
Bran	4
Cinnamon apple	2
English, cinn raisin	2
English, plain	1
English, raisin bran	3

ROLLS

	fat (grams)
Crescent	4
Croissant	12
Hot dog	2
Hamburger	2
Dinner, hard	2
Dinner, soft	3
Kaiser	2
Parker house	2
Submarine	8

fat (grams): 0 10 20 30 40

* Counts are based on single, average-size items. Average
sweet muffin is assumed to be 2 3/4 inches by 2 inches.
Average sweet and English muffin weight is 57 grams.

6

Bread, Crackers, and Flours:
BREAD*

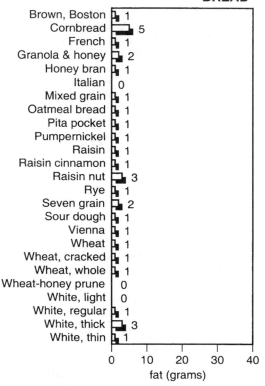

Bread	fat (grams)
Brown, Boston	1
Cornbread	5
French	1
Granola & honey	2
Honey bran	1
Italian	0
Mixed grain	1
Oatmeal bread	1
Pita pocket	1
Pumpernickel	1
Raisin	1
Raisin cinnamon	1
Raisin nut	3
Rye	1
Seven grain	2
Sour dough	1
Vienna	1
Wheat	1
Wheat, cracked	1
Wheat, whole	1
Wheat-honey prune	0
White, light	0
White, regular	1
White, thick	3
White, thin	1

fat (grams)

* Counts are based on single, average-size slices.

7

Bread, Crackers, and Flours:
CRACKERS*

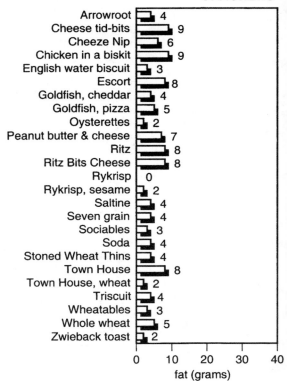

	fat (grams)
Arrowroot	4
Cheese tid-bits	9
Cheeze Nip	6
Chicken in a biskit	9
English water biscuit	3
Escort	8
Goldfish, cheddar	4
Goldfish, pizza	5
Oysterettes	2
Peanut butter & cheese	7
Ritz	8
Ritz Bits Cheese	8
Rykrisp	0
Rykrisp, sesame	2
Saltine	4
Seven grain	4
Sociables	3
Soda	4
Stoned Wheat Thins	4
Town House	8
Town House, wheat	2
Triscuit	4
Wheatables	3
Whole wheat	5
Zwieback toast	2

0   10   20   30   40
fat (grams)

* For ease of comparison, counts are based on one-ounce
servings. Adjust counts to reflect quantities consumed.

Bread, Crackers, and Flours:
DRY & CRISPY*

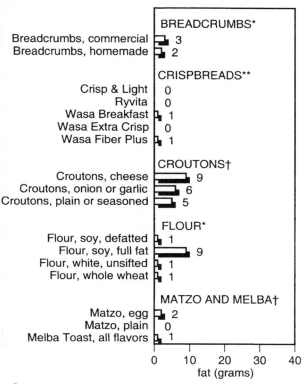

BREADCRUMBS*

Breadcrumbs, commercial — 3
Breadcrumbs, homemade — 2

CRISPBREADS**

Crisp & Light — 0
Ryvita — 0
Wasa Breakfast — 1
Wasa Extra Crisp — 0
Wasa Fiber Plus — 1

CROUTONS†

Croutons, cheese — 9
Croutons, onion or garlic — 6
Croutons, plain or seasoned — 5

FLOUR*

Flour, soy, defatted — 1
Flour, soy, full fat — 9
Flour, white, unsifted — 1
Flour, whole wheat — 1

MATZO AND MELBA†

Matzo, egg — 2
Matzo, plain — 0
Melba Toast, all flavors — 1

0   10   20   30   40
fat (grams)

* Counts are based on 1/2- cup servings.
** Counts are based on single item.
† Counts are based on single-ounce servings.

Bread, Crackers, and Flours:
PANCAKES, STUFFING & MORE*

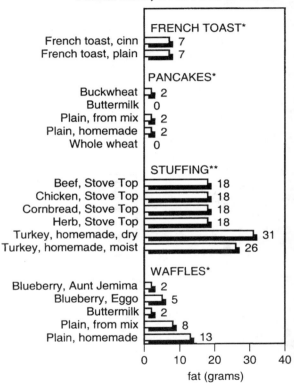

FRENCH TOAST*

French toast, cinn	7
French toast, plain	7

PANCAKES*

Buckwheat	2
Buttermilk	0
Plain, from mix	2
Plain, homemade	2
Whole wheat	0

STUFFING**

Beef, Stove Top	18
Chicken, Stove Top	18
Cornbread, Stove Top	18
Herb, Stove Top	18
Turkey, homemade, dry	31
Turkey, homemade, moist	26

WAFFLES*

Blueberry, Aunt Jemima	2
Blueberry, Eggo	5
Buttermilk	2
Plain, from mix	8
Plain, homemade	13

fat (grams)

*   Counts are based on single slice, pancake, or waffle.
** Counts are based on 1/2-cup servings, prepared.

10

CEREALS*, Part 1

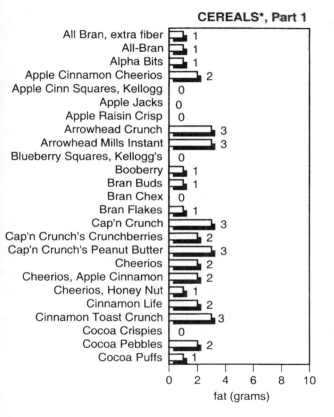

Cereal	fat (grams)
All Bran, extra fiber	1
All-Bran	1
Alpha Bits	1
Apple Cinnamon Cheerios	2
Apple Cinn Squares, Kellogg	0
Apple Jacks	0
Apple Raisin Crisp	0
Arrowhead Crunch	3
Arrowhead Mills Instant	3
Blueberry Squares, Kellogg's	0
Booberry	1
Bran Buds	1
Bran Chex	0
Bran Flakes	1
Cap'n Crunch	3
Cap'n Crunch's Crunchberries	2
Cap'n Crunch's Peanut Butter	3
Cheerios	2
Cheerios, Apple Cinnamon	2
Cheerios, Honey Nut	1
Cinnamon Life	2
Cinnamon Toast Crunch	3
Cocoa Crispies	0
Cocoa Pebbles	2
Cocoa Puffs	1

* Counts are based on average-size servings (as indicated
on package) and without added milk.

11

CEREALS*, Part 2

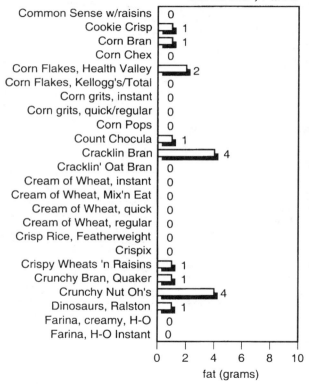

Cereal	fat (grams)
Common Sense w/raisins	0
Cookie Crisp	1
Corn Bran	1
Corn Chex	0
Corn Flakes, Health Valley	2
Corn Flakes, Kellogg's/Total	0
Corn grits, instant	0
Corn grits, quick/regular	0
Corn Pops	0
Count Chocula	1
Cracklin Bran	4
Cracklin' Oat Bran	0
Cream of Wheat, instant	0
Cream of Wheat, Mix'n Eat	0
Cream of Wheat, quick	0
Cream of Wheat, regular	0
Crisp Rice, Featherweight	0
Crispix	0
Crispy Wheats 'n Raisins	1
Crunchy Bran, Quaker	1
Crunchy Nut Oh's	4
Dinosaurs, Ralston	1
Farina, creamy, H-O	0
Farina, H-O Instant	0

* Counts are based on average-size servings (as indicated on package) and without added milk.

CEREALS*, Part 3

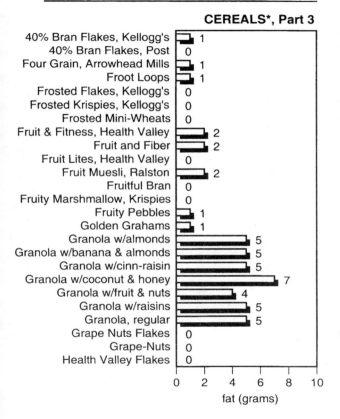

Cereal	fat (grams)
40% Bran Flakes, Kellogg's	1
40% Bran Flakes, Post	0
Four Grain, Arrowhead Mills	1
Froot Loops	1
Frosted Flakes, Kellogg's	0
Frosted Krispies, Kellogg's	0
Frosted Mini-Wheats	0
Fruit & Fitness, Health Valley	2
Fruit and Fiber	2
Fruit Lites, Health Valley	0
Fruit Muesli, Ralston	2
Fruitful Bran	0
Fruity Marshmallow, Krispies	0
Fruity Pebbles	1
Golden Grahams	1
Granola w/almonds	5
Granola w/banana & almonds	5
Granola w/cinn-raisin	5
Granola w/coconut & honey	7
Granola w/fruit & nuts	4
Granola w/raisins	5
Granola, regular	5
Grape Nuts Flakes	0
Grape-Nuts	0
Health Valley Flakes	0

fat (grams)

* Counts are based on average-size servings (as indicated
on package) and without added milk.

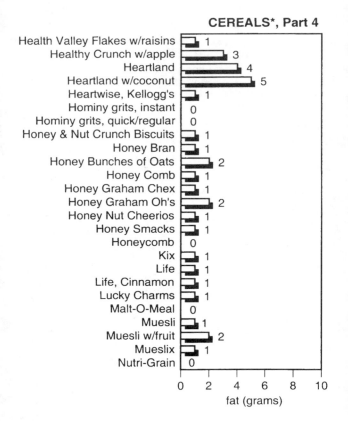

CEREALS*, Part 4

Cereal	fat (grams)
Health Valley Flakes w/raisins	1
Healthy Crunch w/apple	3
Heartland	4
Heartland w/coconut	5
Heartwise, Kellogg's	1
Hominy grits, instant	0
Hominy grits, quick/regular	0
Honey & Nut Crunch Biscuits	1
Honey Bran	1
Honey Bunches of Oats	2
Honey Comb	1
Honey Graham Chex	1
Honey Graham Oh's	2
Honey Nut Cheerios	1
Honey Smacks	1
Honeycomb	0
Kix	1
Life	1
Life, Cinnamon	1
Lucky Charms	1
Malt-O-Meal	0
Muesli	1
Muesli w/fruit	2
Mueslix	1
Nutri-Grain	0

fat (grams)

* Counts are based on average-size servings (as indicated
on package) and without added milk.

Alphabetical Chart
(for Hi-Low Comparison Charts, see pages 83 - 164)

CEREALS*, Part 5

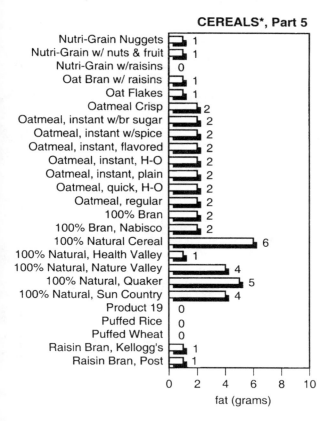

Cereal	fat (grams)
Nutri-Grain Nuggets	1
Nutri-Grain w/ nuts & fruit	1
Nutri-Grain w/raisins	0
Oat Bran w/ raisins	1
Oat Flakes	1
Oatmeal Crisp	2
Oatmeal, instant w/br sugar	2
Oatmeal, instant w/spice	2
Oatmeal, instant, flavored	2
Oatmeal, instant, H-O	2
Oatmeal, instant, plain	2
Oatmeal, quick, H-O	2
Oatmeal, regular	2
100% Bran	2
100% Bran, Nabisco	2
100% Natural Cereal	6
100% Natural, Health Valley	1
100% Natural, Nature Valley	4
100% Natural, Quaker	5
100% Natural, Sun Country	4
Product 19	0
Puffed Rice	0
Puffed Wheat	0
Raisin Bran, Kellogg's	1
Raisin Bran, Post	1

* Counts are based on average-size servings (as indicated
on package) and without added milk.

15

CEREALS, Part 6

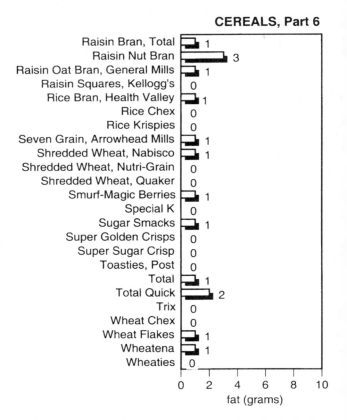

Cereal	fat (grams)
Raisin Bran, Total	1
Raisin Nut Bran	3
Raisin Oat Bran, General Mills	1
Raisin Squares, Kellogg's	0
Rice Bran, Health Valley	1
Rice Chex	0
Rice Krispies	0
Seven Grain, Arrowhead Mills	1
Shredded Wheat, Nabisco	1
Shredded Wheat, Nutri-Grain	0
Shredded Wheat, Quaker	0
Smurf-Magic Berries	1
Special K	0
Sugar Smacks	1
Super Golden Crisps	0
Super Sugar Crisp	0
Toasties, Post	0
Total	1
Total Quick	2
Trix	0
Wheat Chex	0
Wheat Flakes	1
Wheatena	1
Wheaties	0

fat (grams)

* Counts are based on average-size servings (as indicated
on package) and without added milk.

COMBINED AND FROZEN FOODS*,
Part 1

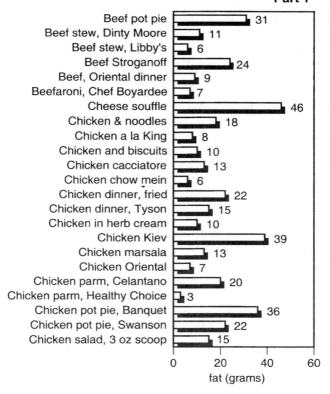

Food	fat (grams)
Beef pot pie	31
Beef stew, Dinty Moore	11
Beef stew, Libby's	6
Beef Stroganoff	24
Beef, Oriental dinner	9
Beefaroni, Chef Boyardee	7
Cheese souffle	46
Chicken & noodles	18
Chicken a la King	8
Chicken and biscuits	10
Chicken cacciatore	13
Chicken chow mein	6
Chicken dinner, fried	22
Chicken dinner, Tyson	15
Chicken in herb cream	10
Chicken Kiev	39
Chicken marsala	13
Chicken Oriental	7
Chicken parm, Celantano	20
Chicken parm, Healthy Choice	3
Chicken pot pie, Banquet	36
Chicken pot pie, Swanson	22
Chicken salad, 3 oz scoop	15

fat (grams): 0   20   40   60

* Counts are based on average-size servings as indicated
on package. Adjust count to reflect amount consumed.

COMBINED AND FROZEN FOODS*,
Part 2

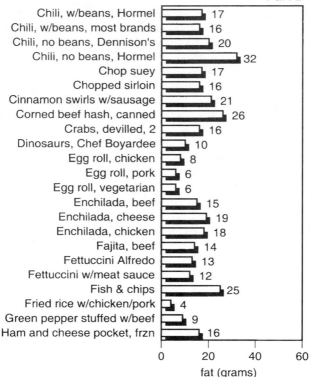

Food	fat (grams)
Chili, w/beans, Hormel	17
Chili, w/beans, most brands	16
Chili, no beans, Dennison's	20
Chili, no beans, Hormel	32
Chop suey	17
Chopped sirloin	16
Cinnamon swirls w/sausage	21
Corned beef hash, canned	26
Crabs, devilled, 2	16
Dinosaurs, Chef Boyardee	10
Egg roll, chicken	8
Egg roll, pork	6
Egg roll, vegetarian	6
Enchilada, beef	15
Enchilada, cheese	19
Enchilada, chicken	18
Fajita, beef	14
Fettuccini Alfredo	13
Fettuccini w/meat sauce	12
Fish & chips	25
Fried rice w/chicken/pork	4
Green pepper stuffed w/beef	9
Ham and cheese pocket, frzn	16

* Counts are based on average-size servings as indicated
on package. Adjust count to reflect amount consumed.

18

COMBINED AND FROZEN FOODS*,
Part 3

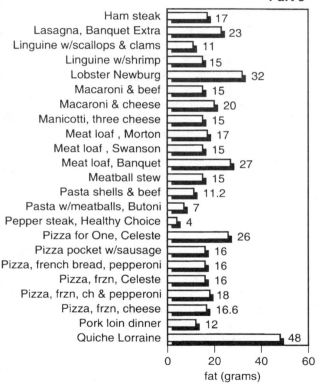

Food	fat (grams)
Ham steak	17
Lasagna, Banquet Extra	23
Linguine w/scallops & clams	11
Linguine w/shrimp	15
Lobster Newburg	32
Macaroni & beef	15
Macaroni & cheese	20
Manicotti, three cheese	15
Meat loaf , Morton	17
Meat loaf , Swanson	15
Meat loaf, Banquet	27
Meatball stew	15
Pasta shells & beef	11.2
Pasta w/meatballs, Butoni	7
Pepper steak, Healthy Choice	4
Pizza for One, Celeste	26
Pizza pocket w/sausage	16
Pizza, french bread, pepperoni	16
Pizza, frzn, Celeste	16
Pizza, frzn, ch & pepperoni	18
Pizza, frzn, cheese	16.6
Pork loin dinner	12
Quiche Lorraine	48

fat (grams)

* Counts are based on average-size servings as indicated
on package. Adjust count to reflect amount consumed.

COMBINED AND FROZEN FOODS*,
Part 4

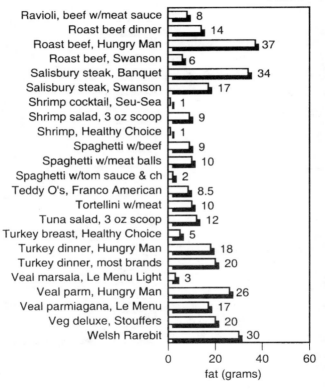

Food	fat (grams)
Ravioli, beef w/meat sauce	8
Roast beef dinner	14
Roast beef, Hungry Man	37
Roast beef, Swanson	6
Salisbury steak, Banquet	34
Salisbury steak, Swanson	17
Shrimp cocktail, Seu-Sea	1
Shrimp salad, 3 oz scoop	9
Shrimp, Healthy Choice	1
Spaghetti w/beef	9
Spaghetti w/meat balls	10
Spaghetti w/tom sauce & ch	2
Teddy O's, Franco American	8.5
Tortellini w/meat	10
Tuna salad, 3 oz scoop	12
Turkey breast, Healthy Choice	5
Turkey dinner, Hungry Man	18
Turkey dinner, most brands	20
Veal marsala, Le Menu Light	3
Veal parm, Hungry Man	26
Veal parmiagana, Le Menu	17
Veg deluxe, Stouffers	20
Welsh Rarebit	30

* Counts are based on average-size servings as indicated
on package. Adjust count to reflect amount consumed.

Dairy: CHEESE (HARD & SEMI-SOFT)*

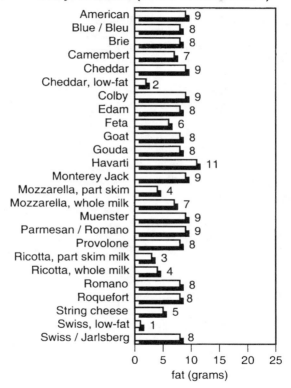

Cheese	fat (grams)
American	9
Blue / Bleu	8
Brie	8
Camembert	7
Cheddar	9
Cheddar, low-fat	2
Colby	9
Edam	8
Feta	6
Goat	8
Gouda	8
Havarti	11
Monterey Jack	9
Mozzarella, part skim	4
Mozzarella, whole milk	7
Muenster	9
Parmesan / Romano	9
Provolone	8
Ricotta, part skim milk	3
Ricotta, whole milk	4
Romano	8
Roquefort	8
String cheese	5
Swiss, low-fat	1
Swiss / Jarlsberg	8

* Counts are based on one-ounce servings. Adjust count
   to reflect amount consumed.

Dairy: CHEESES (SOFT), CREAMS & SUBSTITUTES*

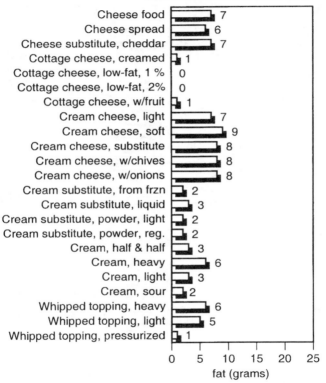

	fat (grams)
Cheese food	7
Cheese spread	6
Cheese substitute, cheddar	7
Cottage cheese, creamed	1
Cottage cheese, low-fat, 1 %	0
Cottage cheese, low-fat, 2%	0
Cottage cheese, w/fruit	1
Cream cheese, light	7
Cream cheese, soft	9
Cream cheese, substitute	8
Cream cheese, w/chives	8
Cream cheese, w/onions	8
Cream substitute, from frzn	2
Cream substitute, liquid	3
Cream substitute, powder, light	2
Cream substitute, powder, reg.	2
Cream, half & half	3
Cream, heavy	6
Cream, light	3
Cream, sour	2
Whipped topping, heavy	6
Whipped topping, light	5
Whipped topping, pressurized	1

* Counts are based on one-ounce servings of soft cheese
or one tablespoon of cream or whipped topping.

Alphabetical Chart
(for Hi-Low Comparison Charts, see pages 83 - 164)

**Dairy: EGGS, MILK,
YOGURT & SHAKES***

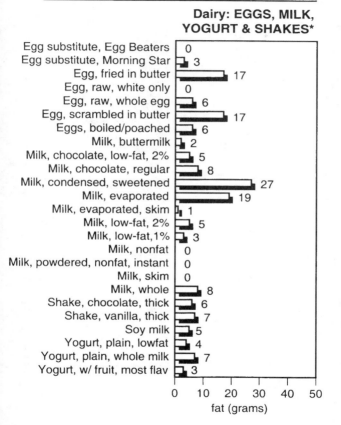

	fat (grams)
Egg substitute, Egg Beaters	0
Egg substitute, Morning Star	3
Egg, fried in butter	17
Egg, raw, white only	0
Egg, raw, whole egg	6
Egg, scrambled in butter	17
Eggs, boiled/poached	6
Milk, buttermilk	2
Milk, chocolate, low-fat, 2%	5
Milk, chocolate, regular	8
Milk, condensed, sweetened	27
Milk, evaporated	19
Milk, evaporated, skim	1
Milk, low-fat, 2%	5
Milk, low-fat,1%	3
Milk, nonfat	0
Milk, powdered, nonfat, instant	0
Milk, skim	0
Milk, whole	8
Shake, chocolate, thick	6
Shake, vanilla, thick	7
Soy milk	5
Yogurt, plain, lowfat	4
Yogurt, plain, whole milk	7
Yogurt, w/ fruit, most flav	3

* Counts based on one egg or equivalent egg substitute or 8 fluid ounces of milk, yogurt, or shake.

Alphabetical Chart
(for Hi-Low Comparison Charts, see pages 83 - 164)

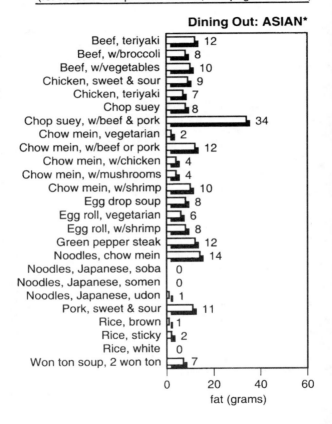

Dining Out: ASIAN*

Food	fat (grams)
Beef, teriyaki	12
Beef, w/broccoli	8
Beef, w/vegetables	10
Chicken, sweet & sour	9
Chicken, teriyaki	7
Chop suey	8
Chop suey, w/beef & pork	34
Chow mein, vegetarian	2
Chow mein, w/beef or pork	12
Chow mein, w/chicken	4
Chow mein, w/mushrooms	4
Chow mein, w/shrimp	10
Egg drop soup	8
Egg roll, vegetarian	6
Egg roll, w/shrimp	8
Green pepper steak	12
Noodles, chow mein	14
Noodles, Japanese, soba	0
Noodles, Japanese, somen	0
Noodles, Japanese, udon	1
Pork, sweet & sour	11
Rice, brown	1
Rice, sticky	2
Rice, white	0
Won ton soup, 2 won ton	7

* Counts based on average-sized servings (for main dishes,
1 1/2 - 2 cups). Counts for main dishes include rice.

24

Dining Out: DELICATESSEN*

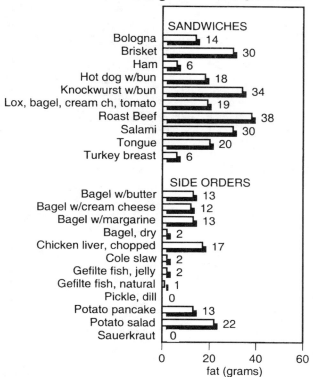

SANDWICHES

Bologna	14
Brisket	30
Ham	6
Hot dog w/bun	18
Knockwurst w/bun	34
Lox, bagel, cream ch, tomato	19
Roast Beef	38
Salami	30
Tongue	20
Turkey breast	6

SIDE ORDERS

Bagel w/butter	13
Bagel w/cream cheese	12
Bagel w/margarine	13
Bagel, dry	2
Chicken liver, chopped	17
Cole slaw	2
Gefilte fish, jelly	2
Gefilte fish, natural	1
Pickle, dill	0
Potato pancake	13
Potato salad	22
Sauerkraut	0

0   20   40   60
fat (grams)

* Unless otherwise indicated, counts based on average-
size servings or sandwiches. Sandwich counts assume
white or rye bread.

Dining Out: FRENCH AND OTHER INTERNATIONAL DISHES*

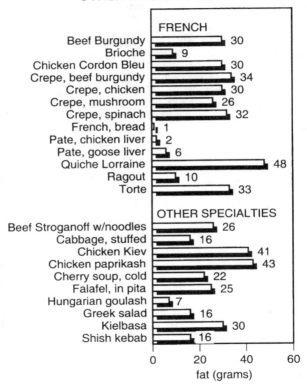

FRENCH

Dish	fat (grams)
Beef Burgundy	30
Brioche	9
Chicken Cordon Bleu	30
Crepe, beef burgundy	34
Crepe, chicken	30
Crepe, mushroom	26
Crepe, spinach	32
French, bread	1
Pate, chicken liver	2
Pate, goose liver	6
Quiche Lorraine	48
Ragout	10
Torte	33

OTHER SPECIALTIES

Dish	fat (grams)
Beef Stroganoff w/noodles	26
Cabbage, stuffed	16
Chicken Kiev	41
Chicken paprikash	43
Cherry soup, cold	22
Falafel, in pita	25
Hungarian goulash	7
Greek salad	16
Kielbasa	30
Shish kebab	16

fat (grams)

* Counts based on average-sized servings (for main dishes,
1 1/2 - 2 cups).

Dining Out: ITALIAN*

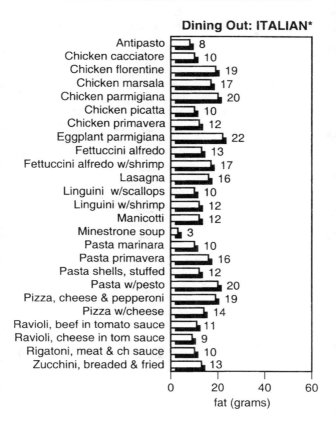

Food	fat (grams)
Antipasto	8
Chicken cacciatore	10
Chicken florentine	19
Chicken marsala	17
Chicken parmigiana	20
Chicken picatta	10
Chicken primavera	12
Eggplant parmigiana	22
Fettuccini alfredo	13
Fettuccini alfredo w/shrimp	17
Lasagna	16
Linguini w/scallops	10
Linguini w/shrimp	12
Manicotti	12
Minestrone soup	3
Pasta marinara	10
Pasta primavera	16
Pasta shells, stuffed	12
Pasta w/pesto	20
Pizza, cheese & pepperoni	19
Pizza w/cheese	14
Ravioli, beef in tomato sauce	11
Ravioli, cheese in tom sauce	9
Rigatoni, meat & ch sauce	10
Zucchini, breaded & fried	13

fat (grams) — 0 20 40 60

* Counts are based on average-sized servings (1 1/2 - 2 cups); for pizza, on 1/6 medium or 1/8 large pizza).

Dining Out: MEXICAN*

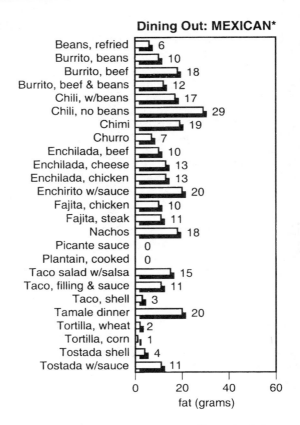

	fat (grams)
Beans, refried	6
Burrito, beans	10
Burrito, beef	18
Burrito, beef & beans	12
Chili, w/beans	17
Chili, no beans	29
Chimi	19
Churro	7
Enchilada, beef	10
Enchilada, cheese	13
Enchilada, chicken	13
Enchirito w/sauce	20
Fajita, chicken	10
Fajita, steak	11
Nachos	18
Picante sauce	0
Plantain, cooked	0
Taco salad w/salsa	15
Taco, filling & sauce	11
Taco, shell	3
Tamale dinner	20
Tortilla, wheat	2
Tortilla, corn	1
Tostada shell	4
Tostada w/sauce	11

* Counts based on average-sized servings (for main dishes,
1 1/2 - 2 cups).

Alphabetical Chart
(for Hi-Low Comparison Charts, see pages 83 - 164)

Fast Food: ARBY'S*

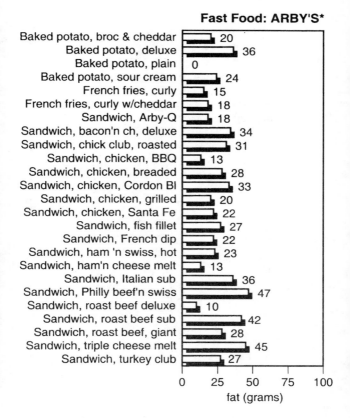

	fat (grams)
Baked potato, broc & cheddar	20
Baked potato, deluxe	36
Baked potato, plain	0
Baked potato, sour cream	24
French fries, curly	15
French fries, curly w/cheddar	18
Sandwich, Arby-Q	18
Sandwich, bacon'n ch, deluxe	34
Sandwich, chick club, roasted	31
Sandwich, chicken, BBQ	13
Sandwich, chicken, breaded	28
Sandwich, chicken, Cordon Bl	33
Sandwich, chicken, grilled	20
Sandwich, chicken, Santa Fe	22
Sandwich, fish fillet	27
Sandwich, French dip	22
Sandwich, ham 'n swiss, hot	23
Sandwich, ham'n cheese melt	13
Sandwich, Italian sub	36
Sandwich, Philly beef'n swiss	47
Sandwich, roast beef deluxe	10
Sandwich, roast beef sub	42
Sandwich, roast beef, giant	28
Sandwich, triple cheese melt	45
Sandwich, turkey club	27

fat (grams)

* Unless otherwise indicated, counts are based on average-
size servings.

Fast Food: BOSTON MARKET*

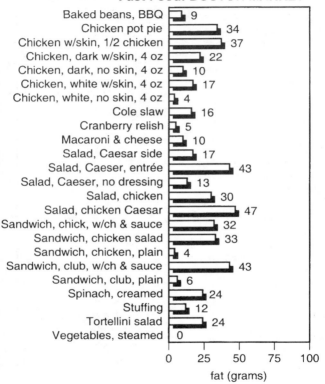

Food	fat (grams)
Baked beans, BBQ	9
Chicken pot pie	34
Chicken w/skin, 1/2 chicken	37
Chicken, dark w/skin, 4 oz	22
Chicken, dark, no skin, 4 oz	10
Chicken, white w/skin, 4 oz	17
Chicken, white, no skin, 4 oz	4
Cole slaw	16
Cranberry relish	5
Macaroni & cheese	10
Salad, Caesar side	17
Salad, Caeser, entrée	43
Salad, Caeser, no dressing	13
Salad, chicken	30
Salad, chicken Caesar	47
Sandwich, chick, w/ch & sauce	32
Sandwich, chicken salad	33
Sandwich, chicken, plain	4
Sandwich, club, w/ch & sauce	43
Sandwich, club, plain	6
Spinach, creamed	24
Stuffing	12
Tortellini salad	24
Vegetables, steamed	0

* Unless otherwise indicated, counts are based on average-size servings.

30

Fast Food: BURGER KING*

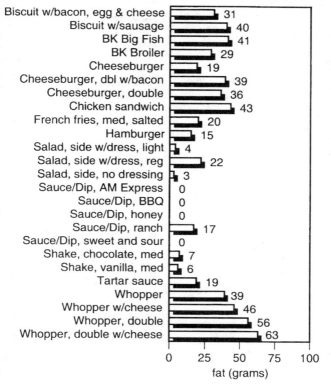

Item	fat (grams)
Biscuit w/bacon, egg & cheese	31
Biscuit w/sausage	40
BK Big Fish	41
BK Broiler	29
Cheeseburger	19
Cheeseburger, dbl w/bacon	39
Cheeseburger, double	36
Chicken sandwich	43
French fries, med, salted	20
Hamburger	15
Salad, side w/dress, light	4
Salad, side w/dress, reg	22
Salad, side, no dressing	3
Sauce/Dip, AM Express	0
Sauce/Dip, BBQ	0
Sauce/Dip, honey	0
Sauce/Dip, ranch	17
Sauce/Dip, sweet and sour	0
Shake, chocolate, med	7
Shake, vanilla, med	6
Tartar sauce	19
Whopper	39
Whopper w/cheese	46
Whopper, double	56
Whopper, double w/cheese	63

* Unless otherwise indicated, counts are based on average-size servings.

Fast Food: HARDEE'S*

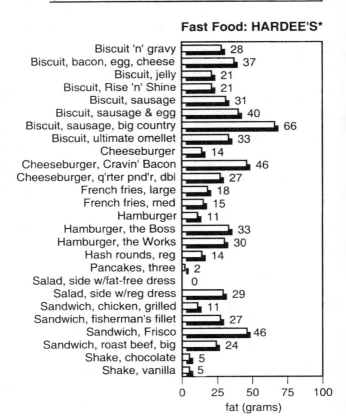

Item	fat (grams)
Biscuit 'n' gravy	28
Biscuit, bacon, egg, cheese	37
Biscuit, jelly	21
Biscuit, Rise 'n' Shine	21
Biscuit, sausage	31
Biscuit, sausage & egg	40
Biscuit, sausage, big country	66
Biscuit, ultimate omelet	33
Cheeseburger	14
Cheeseburger, Cravin' Bacon	46
Cheeseburger, q'rter pnd'r, dbl	27
French fries, large	18
French fries, med	15
Hamburger	11
Hamburger, the Boss	33
Hamburger, the Works	30
Hash rounds, reg	14
Pancakes, three	2
Salad, side w/fat-free dress	0
Salad, side w/reg dress	29
Sandwich, chicken, grilled	11
Sandwich, fisherman's fillet	27
Sandwich, Frisco	46
Sandwich, roast beef, big	24
Shake, chocolate	5
Shake, vanilla	5

* Unless otherwise indicated, counts are based on average-size servings.

32

Fast Food: JACK IN THE BOX*

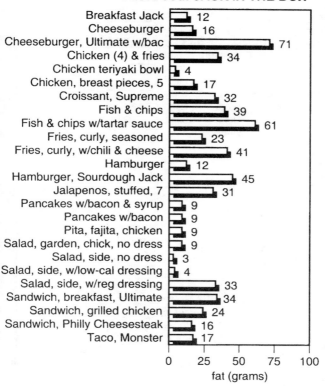

Food	fat (grams)
Breakfast Jack	12
Cheeseburger	16
Cheeseburger, Ultimate w/bac	71
Chicken (4) & fries	34
Chicken teriyaki bowl	4
Chicken, breast pieces, 5	17
Croissant, Supreme	32
Fish & chips	39
Fish & chips w/tartar sauce	61
Fries, curly, seasoned	23
Fries, curly, w/chili & cheese	41
Hamburger	12
Hamburger, Sourdough Jack	45
Jalapenos, stuffed, 7	31
Pancakes w/bacon & syrup	9
Pancakes w/bacon	9
Pita, fajita, chicken	9
Salad, garden, chick, no dress	9
Salad, side, no dress	3
Salad, side, w/low-cal dressing	4
Salad, side, w/reg dressing	33
Sandwich, breakfast, Ultimate	34
Sandwich, grilled chicken	24
Sandwich, Philly Cheesesteak	16
Taco, Monster	17

* Unless otherwise indicated, counts are based on average-size servings.

Fast Food: KFC*

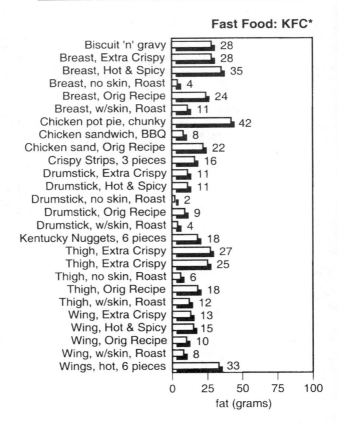

Item	fat (grams)
Biscuit 'n' gravy	28
Breast, Extra Crispy	28
Breast, Hot & Spicy	35
Breast, no skin, Roast	4
Breast, Orig Recipe	24
Breast, w/skin, Roast	11
Chicken pot pie, chunky	42
Chicken sandwich, BBQ	8
Chicken sand, Orig Recipe	22
Crispy Strips, 3 pieces	16
Drumstick, Extra Crispy	11
Drumstick, Hot & Spicy	11
Drumstick, no skin, Roast	2
Drumstick, Orig Recipe	9
Drumstick, w/skin, Roast	4
Kentucky Nuggets, 6 pieces	18
Thigh, Extra Crispy	27
Thigh, Extra Crispy	25
Thigh, no skin, Roast	6
Thigh, Orig Recipe	18
Thigh, w/skin, Roast	12
Wing, Extra Crispy	13
Wing, Hot & Spicy	15
Wing, Orig Recipe	10
Wing, w/skin, Roast	8
Wings, hot, 6 pieces	33

fat (grams)

* Unless otherwise indicated, counts are based on average-size servings.

Fast Food: MC DONALD'S*

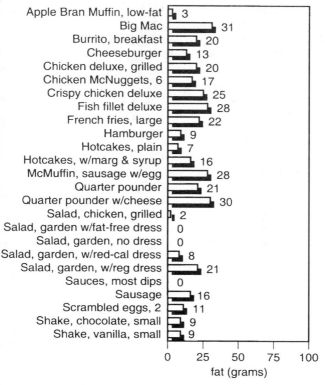

Food	fat (grams)
Apple Bran Muffin, low-fat	3
Big Mac	31
Burrito, breakfast	20
Cheeseburger	13
Chicken deluxe, grilled	20
Chicken McNuggets, 6	17
Crispy chicken deluxe	25
Fish fillet deluxe	28
French fries, large	22
Hamburger	9
Hotcakes, plain	7
Hotcakes, w/marg & syrup	16
McMuffin, sausage w/egg	28
Quarter pounder	21
Quarter pounder w/cheese	30
Salad, chicken, grilled	2
Salad, garden w/fat-free dress	0
Salad, garden, no dress	0
Salad, garden, w/red-cal dress	8
Salad, garden, w/reg dress	21
Sauces, most dips	0
Sausage	16
Scrambled eggs, 2	11
Shake, chocolate, small	9
Shake, vanilla, small	9

fat (grams)

* Unless otherwise indicated, counts are based on average-size servings.

35

Fast Food: PIZZA HUT*

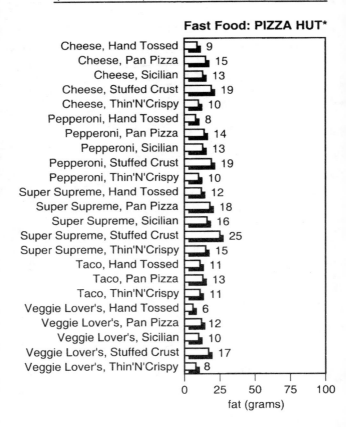

	fat (grams)
Cheese, Hand Tossed	9
Cheese, Pan Pizza	15
Cheese, Sicilian	13
Cheese, Stuffed Crust	19
Cheese, Thin'N'Crispy	10
Pepperoni, Hand Tossed	8
Pepperoni, Pan Pizza	14
Pepperoni, Sicilian	13
Pepperoni, Stuffed Crust	19
Pepperoni, Thin'N'Crispy	10
Super Supreme, Hand Tossed	12
Super Supreme, Pan Pizza	18
Super Supreme, Sicilian	16
Super Supreme, Stuffed Crust	25
Super Supreme, Thin'N'Crispy	15
Taco, Hand Tossed	11
Taco, Pan Pizza	13
Taco, Thin'N'Crispy	11
Veggie Lover's, Hand Tossed	6
Veggie Lover's, Pan Pizza	12
Veggie Lover's, Sicilian	10
Veggie Lover's, Stuffed Crust	17
Veggie Lover's, Thin'N'Crispy	8

* Unless otherwise indicated, counts are based on average-size servings.

36

Fast Food: SUBWAY*

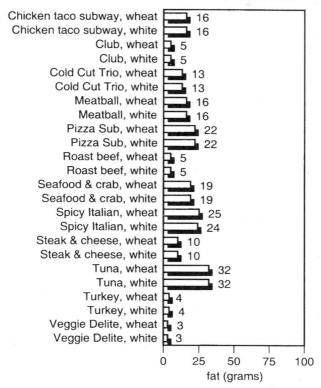

Item	fat (grams)
Chicken taco subway, wheat	16
Chicken taco subway, white	16
Club, wheat	5
Club, white	5
Cold Cut Trio, wheat	13
Cold Cut Trio, white	13
Meatball, wheat	16
Meatball, white	16
Pizza Sub, wheat	22
Pizza Sub, white	22
Roast beef, wheat	5
Roast beef, white	5
Seafood & crab, wheat	19
Seafood & crab, white	19
Spicy Italian, wheat	25
Spicy Italian, white	24
Steak & cheese, wheat	10
Steak & cheese, white	10
Tuna, wheat	32
Tuna, white	32
Turkey, wheat	4
Turkey, white	4
Veggie Delite, wheat	3
Veggie Delite, white	3

fat (grams)

* Unless otherwise indicated, counts are based on average-size servings.

Fast Food: TACO BELL*

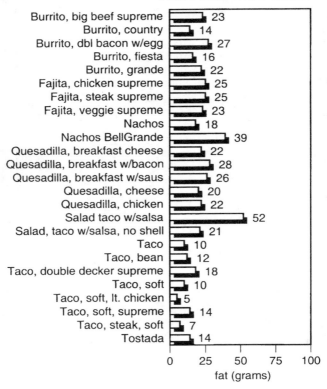

Item	fat (grams)
Burrito, big beef supreme	23
Burrito, country	14
Burrito, dbl bacon w/egg	27
Burrito, fiesta	16
Burrito, grande	22
Fajita, chicken supreme	25
Fajita, steak supreme	25
Fajita, veggie supreme	23
Nachos	18
Nachos BellGrande	39
Quesadilla, breakfast cheese	22
Quesadilla, breakfast w/bacon	28
Quesadilla, breakfast w/saus	26
Quesadilla, cheese	20
Quesadilla, chicken	22
Salad taco w/salsa	52
Salad, taco w/salsa, no shell	21
Taco	10
Taco, bean	12
Taco, double decker supreme	18
Taco, soft	10
Taco, soft, lt. chicken	5
Taco, soft, supreme	14
Taco, steak, soft	7
Tostada	14

fat (grams)

* Unless otherwise indicated, counts are based on average-size servings.

38

Fast Food: WENDY'S*

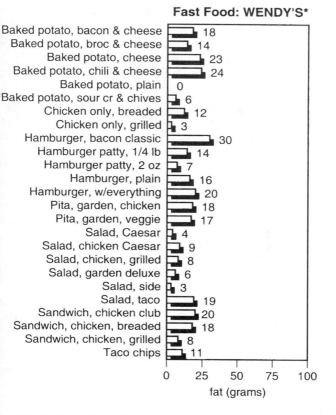

Food	fat (grams)
Baked potato, bacon & cheese	18
Baked potato, broc & cheese	14
Baked potato, cheese	23
Baked potato, chili & cheese	24
Baked potato, plain	0
Baked potato, sour cr & chives	6
Chicken only, breaded	12
Chicken only, grilled	3
Hamburger, bacon classic	30
Hamburger patty, 1/4 lb	14
Hamburger patty, 2 oz	7
Hamburger, plain	16
Hamburger, w/everything	20
Pita, garden, chicken	18
Pita, garden, veggie	17
Salad, Caesar	4
Salad, chicken Caesar	9
Salad, chicken, grilled	8
Salad, garden deluxe	6
Salad, side	3
Salad, taco	19
Sandwich, chicken club	20
Sandwich, chicken, breaded	18
Sandwich, chicken, grilled	8
Taco chips	11

fat (grams)

* Unless otherwise indicated, counts are based on average-size servings.

Fruits: FRESH & DRIED FRUITS AND JUICES *, Part 1

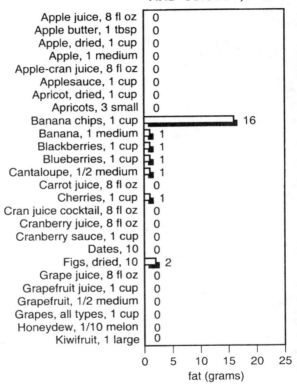

Food	fat (grams)
Apple juice, 8 fl oz	0
Apple butter, 1 tbsp	0
Apple, dried, 1 cup	0
Apple, 1 medium	0
Apple-cran juice, 8 fl oz	0
Applesauce, 1 cup	0
Apricot, dried, 1 cup	0
Apricots, 3 small	0
Banana chips, 1 cup	16
Banana, 1 medium	1
Blackberries, 1 cup	1
Blueberries, 1 cup	1
Cantaloupe, 1/2 medium	1
Carrot juice, 8 fl oz	0
Cherries, 1 cup	1
Cran juice cocktail, 8 fl oz	0
Cranberry juice, 8 fl oz	0
Cranberry sauce, 1 cup	0
Dates, 10	0
Figs, dried, 10	2
Grape juice, 8 fl oz	0
Grapefruit juice, 1 cup	0
Grapefruit, 1/2 medium	0
Grapes, all types, 1 cup	0
Honeydew, 1/10 melon	0
Kiwifruit, 1 large	0

fat (grams)

* Unless otherwise indicated, counts are based on whole, fresh fruits.

40

Fruits: FRESH & DRIED FRUITS
AND JUICES *, Part 2

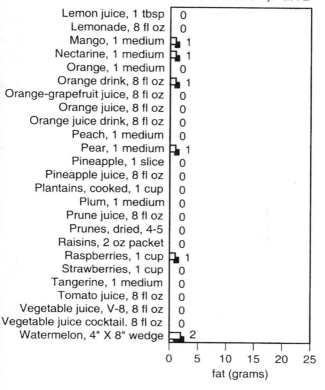

	fat (grams)
Lemon juice, 1 tbsp	0
Lemonade, 8 fl oz	0
Mango, 1 medium	1
Nectarine, 1 medium	1
Orange, 1 medium	0
Orange drink, 8 fl oz	1
Orange-grapefruit juice, 8 fl oz	0
Orange juice, 8 fl oz	0
Orange juice drink, 8 fl oz	0
Peach, 1 medium	0
Pear, 1 medium	1
Pineapple, 1 slice	0
Pineapple juice, 8 fl oz	0
Plantains, cooked, 1 cup	0
Plum, 1 medium	0
Prune juice, 8 fl oz	0
Prunes, dried, 4-5	0
Raisins, 2 oz packet	0
Raspberries, 1 cup	1
Strawberries, 1 cup	0
Tangerine, 1 medium	0
Tomato juice, 8 fl oz	0
Vegetable juice, V-8, 8 fl oz	0
Vegetable juice cocktail. 8 fl oz	0
Watermelon, 4" X 8" wedge	2

0   5   10   15   20   25
fat (grams)

* Unless otherwise indicated, counts are based on whole,
fresh fruits.

GRAVIES, SAUCES & DIPS*

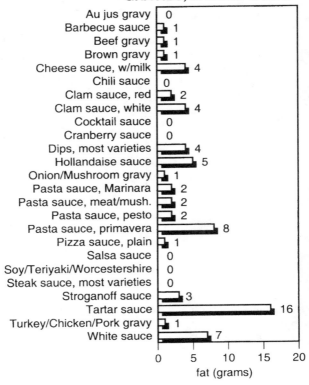

	fat (grams)
Au jus gravy	0
Barbecue sauce	1
Beef gravy	1
Brown gravy	1
Cheese sauce, w/milk	4
Chili sauce	0
Clam sauce, red	2
Clam sauce, white	4
Cocktail sauce	0
Cranberry sauce	0
Dips, most varieties	4
Hollandaise sauce	5
Onion/Mushroom gravy	1
Pasta sauce, Marinara	2
Pasta sauce, meat/mush.	2
Pasta sauce, pesto	2
Pasta sauce, primavera	8
Pizza sauce, plain	1
Salsa sauce	0
Soy/Teriyaki/Worcestershire	0
Steak sauce, most varieties	0
Stroganoff sauce	3
Tartar sauce	16
Turkey/Chicken/Pork gravy	1
White sauce	7

*Counts are based on one-quarter cup servings.

MEATS*, Part 1

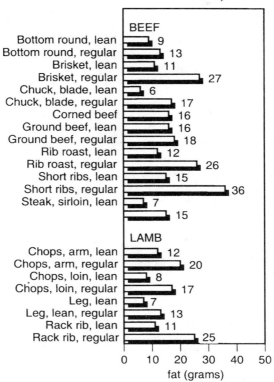

BEEF

Bottom round, lean — 9
Bottom round, regular — 13
Brisket, lean — 11
Brisket, regular — 27
Chuck, blade, lean — 6
Chuck, blade, regular — 17
Corned beef — 16
Ground beef, lean — 16
Ground beef, regular — 18
Rib roast, lean — 12
Rib roast, regular — 26
Short ribs, lean — 15
Short ribs, regular — 36
Steak, sirloin, lean — 7
— 15

LAMB

Chops, arm, lean — 12
Chops, arm, regular — 20
Chops, loin, lean — 8
Chops, loin, regular — 17
Leg, lean — 7
Leg, lean, regular — 13
Rack rib, lean — 11
Rack rib, regular — 25

0   10   20   30   40   50
fat (grams)

* Counts are based on 3-ounce servings.

MEATS*, Part 2

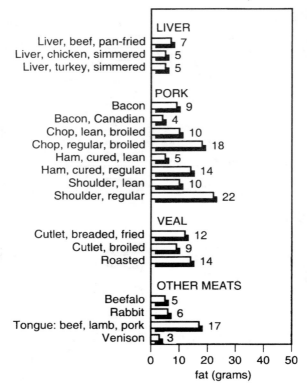

LIVER
- Liver, beef, pan-fried — 7
- Liver, chicken, simmered — 5
- Liver, turkey, simmered — 5

PORK
- Bacon — 9
- Bacon, Canadian — 4
- Chop, lean, broiled — 10
- Chop, regular, broiled — 18
- Ham, cured, lean — 5
- Ham, cured, regular — 14
- Shoulder, lean — 10
- Shoulder, regular — 22

VEAL
- Cutlet, breaded, fried — 12
- Cutlet, broiled — 9
- Roasted — 14

OTHER MEATS
- Beefalo — 5
- Rabbit — 6
- Tongue: beef, lamb, pork — 17
- Venison — 3

0 10 20 30 40 50
fat (grams)

* Counts are based on 3-ounce servings.

MEATS, PROCESSED*

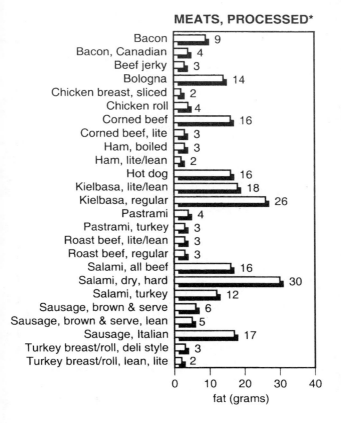

Food	fat (grams)
Bacon	9
Bacon, Canadian	4
Beef jerky	3
Bologna	14
Chicken breast, sliced	2
Chicken roll	4
Corned beef	16
Corned beef, lite	3
Ham, boiled	3
Ham, lite/lean	2
Hot dog	16
Kielbasa, lite/lean	18
Kielbasa, regular	26
Pastrami	4
Pastrami, turkey	3
Roast beef, lite/lean	3
Roast beef, regular	3
Salami, all beef	16
Salami, dry, hard	30
Salami, turkey	12
Sausage, brown & serve	6
Sausage, brown & serve, lean	5
Sausage, Italian	17
Turkey breast/roll, deli style	3
Turkey breast/roll, lean, lite	2

* Counts are based on 3-ounce servings.

Medications: COUGH DROPS & SYRUPS*

	COUGH DROPS
Black, Beech-Nut	0
Cherry, Hall's	0
Cough suppress. lozenges	0
Decongestant lozenges	0
Honey, Pine Brothers	0
Lemon, Hall's	0
Listerine Throat Lozenges	0
Mentho-Lyptus, Hall's	0
Menthol, Beech-Nut	0
Spec T Throat Anesthetic	0
Wild Cherry, Beech-Nut	0
	0
	COUGH SYRUPS
Actifed	0
Comtrex	0
CoTylenol	0
Extra-Strength Tylenol	0
Sudafed	0
Triaminic Expectorant	0
Triaminic Expectorant DH	0
Triaminic Syrup	0

```
0    5    10   15   20   25
            fat (grams)
```

* Counts are based on one cough drop or on recommended
  doses for adults.

Medications: OVER-THE-COUNTER REMEDIES & VITAMINS AND MINERALS*

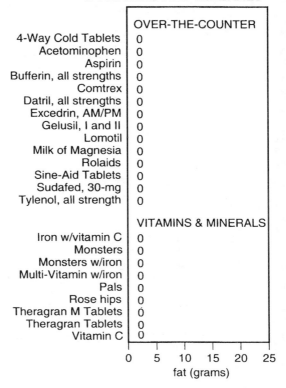

	OVER-THE-COUNTER
4-Way Cold Tablets	0
Acetaminophen	0
Aspirin	0
Bufferin, all strengths	0
Comtrex	0
Datril, all strengths	0
Excedrin, AM/PM	0
Gelusil, I and II	0
Lomotil	0
Milk of Magnesia	0
Rolaids	0
Sine-Aid Tablets	0
Sudafed, 30-mg	0
Tylenol, all strength	0
	VITAMINS & MINERALS
Iron w/vitamin C	0
Monsters	0
Monsters w/iron	0
Multi-Vitamin w/iron	0
Pals	0
Rose hips	0
Theragran M Tablets	0
Theragran Tablets	0
Vitamin C	0

0   5   10   15   20   25
fat (grams)

* Counts are based on recommended doses for adults.

Alphabetical Chart
(for Hi-Low Comparison Charts, see pages 83 - 164)

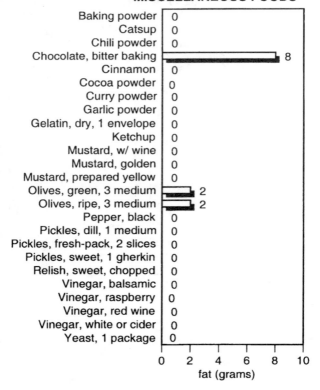

MISCELLANEOUS FOODS*

Food	fat (grams)
Baking powder	0
Catsup	0
Chili powder	0
Chocolate, bitter baking	8
Cinnamon	0
Cocoa powder	0
Curry powder	0
Garlic powder	0
Gelatin, dry, 1 envelope	0
Ketchup	0
Mustard, w/ wine	0
Mustard, golden	0
Mustard, prepared yellow	0
Olives, green, 3 medium	2
Olives, ripe, 3 medium	2
Pepper, black	0
Pickles, dill, 1 medium	0
Pickles, fresh-pack, 2 slices	0
Pickles, sweet, 1 gherkin	0
Relish, sweet, chopped	0
Vinegar, balsamic	0
Vinegar, raspberry	0
Vinegar, red wine	0
Vinegar, white or cider	0
Yeast, 1 package	0

* Unless otherwise indicated, counts are based on
a one-tablespoon serving.

48

NUTS, BEANS AND SEEDS*: Part 1

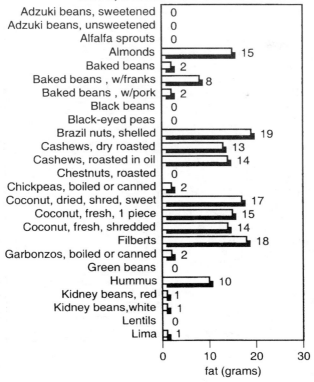

	fat (grams)
Adzuki beans, sweetened	0
Adzuki beans, unsweetened	0
Alfalfa sprouts	0
Almonds	15
Baked beans	2
Baked beans , w/franks	8
Baked beans , w/pork	2
Black beans	0
Black-eyed peas	0
Brazil nuts, shelled	19
Cashews, dry roasted	13
Cashews, roasted in oil	14
Chestnuts, roasted	0
Chickpeas, boiled or canned	2
Coconut, dried, shred, sweet	17
Coconut, fresh, 1 piece	15
Coconut, fresh, shredded	14
Filberts	18
Garbonzos, boiled or canned	2
Green beans	0
Hummus	10
Kidney beans, red	1
Kidney beans,white	1
Lentils	0
Lima	1

* Unless otherwise indicated, counts are based on 1/2 cup
tofu or cooked beans or one-ounce servings of raw nuts or
seeds.

NUTS, BEANS AND SEEDS*: Part 2

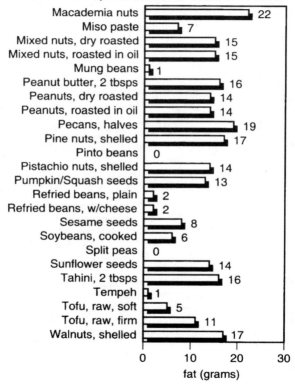

Food	fat (grams)
Macadamia nuts	22
Miso paste	7
Mixed nuts, dry roasted	15
Mixed nuts, roasted in oil	15
Mung beans	1
Peanut butter, 2 tbsps	16
Peanuts, dry roasted	14
Peanuts, roasted in oil	14
Pecans, halves	19
Pine nuts, shelled	17
Pinto beans	0
Pistachio nuts, shelled	14
Pumpkin/Squash seeds	13
Refried beans, plain	2
Refried beans, w/cheese	2
Sesame seeds	8
Soybeans, cooked	6
Split peas	0
Sunflower seeds	14
Tahini, 2 tbsps	16
Tempeh	1
Tofu, raw, soft	5
Tofu, raw, firm	11
Walnuts, shelled	17

* Unless otherwise indicated, counts are based on 1/2 cup tofu or cooked beans or one-ounce servings of raw nuts or seeds.

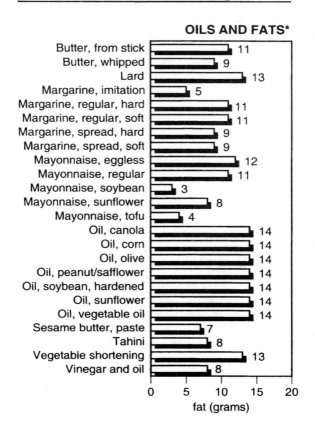

OILS AND FATS*

Item	fat (grams)
Butter, from stick	11
Butter, whipped	9
Lard	13
Margarine, imitation	5
Margarine, regular, hard	11
Margarine, regular, soft	11
Margarine, spread, hard	9
Margarine, spread, soft	9
Mayonnaise, eggless	12
Mayonnaise, regular	11
Mayonnaise, soybean	3
Mayonnaise, sunflower	8
Mayonnaise, tofu	4
Oil, canola	14
Oil, corn	14
Oil, olive	14
Oil, peanut/safflower	14
Oil, soybean, hardened	14
Oil, sunflower	14
Oil, vegetable oil	14
Sesame butter, paste	7
Tahini	8
Vegetable shortening	13
Vinegar and oil	8

* Counts are based on 1-tablespoon servings.

51

PASTA, WHOLE GRAINS , RICE & NOODLES*, Part 1

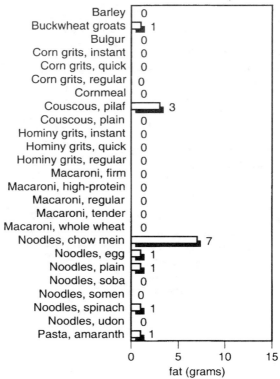

	fat (grams)
Barley	0
Buckwheat groats	1
Bulgur	0
Corn grits, instant	0
Corn grits, quick	0
Corn grits, regular	0
Cornmeal	0
Couscous, pilaf	3
Couscous, plain	0
Hominy grits, instant	0
Hominy grits, quick	0
Hominy grits, regular	0
Macaroni, firm	0
Macaroni, high-protein	0
Macaroni, regular	0
Macaroni, tender	0
Macaroni, whole wheat	0
Noodles, chow mein	7
Noodles, egg	1
Noodles, plain	1
Noodles, soba	0
Noodles, somen	0
Noodles, spinach	1
Noodles, udon	0
Pasta, amaranth	1

* Counts are based on cooked, 1/2-cup servings.

52

**PASTA, WHOLE GRAINS ,
RICE & NOODLES*, Part 2**

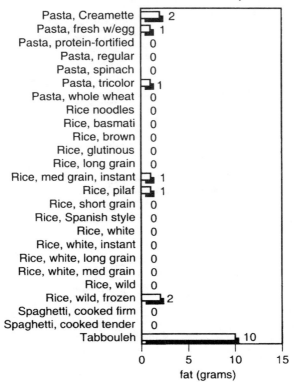

	fat (grams)
Pasta, Creamette	2
Pasta, fresh w/egg	1
Pasta, protein-fortified	0
Pasta, regular	0
Pasta, spinach	0
Pasta, tricolor	1
Pasta, whole wheat	0
Rice noodles	0
Rice, basmati	0
Rice, brown	0
Rice, glutinous	0
Rice, long grain	0
Rice, med grain, instant	1
Rice, pilaf	1
Rice, short grain	0
Rice, Spanish style	0
Rice, white	0
Rice, white, instant	0
Rice, white, long grain	0
Rice, white, med grain	0
Rice, wild	0
Rice, wild, frozen	2
Spaghetti, cooked firm	0
Spaghetti, cooked tender	0
Tabbouleh	10

* Counts are based on cooked, 1/2-cup servings.

Poultry: CHICKEN, TURKEY, AND OTHER FOWL*

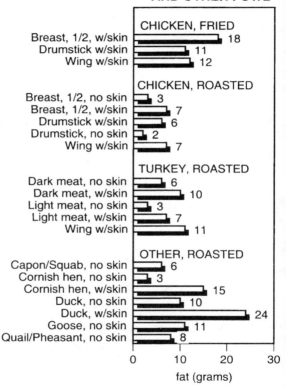

CHICKEN, FRIED
- Breast, 1/2, w/skin — 18
- Drumstick w/skin — 11
- Wing w/skin — 12

CHICKEN, ROASTED
- Breast, 1/2, no skin — 3
- Breast, 1/2, w/skin — 7
- Drumstick w/skin — 6
- Drumstick, no skin — 2
- Wing w/skin — 7

TURKEY, ROASTED
- Dark meat, no skin — 6
- Dark meat, w/skin — 10
- Light meat, no skin — 3
- Light meat, w/skin — 7
- Wing w/skin — 11

OTHER, ROASTED
- Capon/Squab, no skin — 6
- Cornish hen, no skin — 3
- Cornish hen, w/skin — 15
- Duck, no skin — 10
- Duck, w/skin — 24
- Goose, no skin — 11
- Quail/Pheasant, no skin — 8

fat (grams)

* Unless otherwise indicated, counts are based on 3-ounce servings.

54

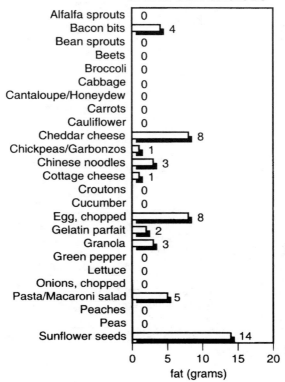

SALAD BAR CHOICES*

*Counts are based on one-quarter cup servings.

SALAD DRESSING*

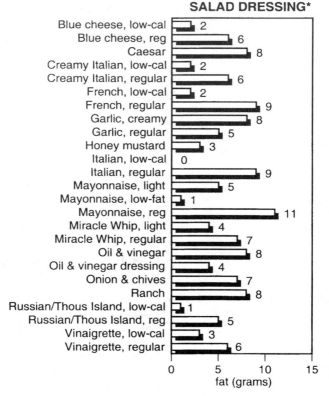

Dressing	fat (grams)
Blue cheese, low-cal	2
Blue cheese, reg	6
Caesar	8
Creamy Italian, low-cal	2
Creamy Italian, regular	6
French, low-cal	2
French, regular	9
Garlic, creamy	8
Garlic, regular	5
Honey mustard	3
Italian, low-cal	0
Italian, regular	9
Mayonnaise, light	5
Mayonnaise, low-fat	1
Mayonnaise, reg	11
Miracle Whip, light	4
Miracle Whip, regular	7
Oil & vinegar	8
Oil & vinegar dressing	4
Onion & chives	7
Ranch	8
Russian/Thous Island, low-cal	1
Russian/Thous Island, reg	5
Vinaigrette, low-cal	3
Vinaigrette, regular	6

* For ease of comparison, counts are based on single
tablespoon servings. Adjust counts to reflect quantities
consumed.

Alphabetical Chart
(for Hi-Low Comparison Charts, see pages 83 - 164)

SEAFOOD*, Part 1

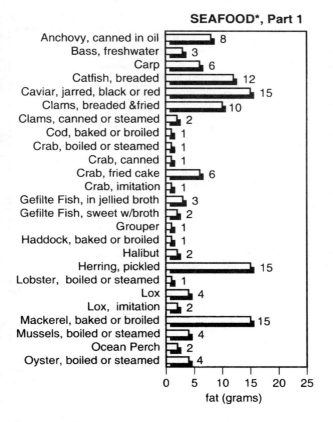

Food	fat (grams)
Anchovy, canned in oil	8
Bass, freshwater	3
Carp	6
Catfish, breaded	12
Caviar, jarred, black or red	15
Clams, breaded &fried	10
Clams, canned or steamed	2
Cod, baked or broiled	1
Crab, boiled or steamed	1
Crab, canned	1
Crab, fried cake	6
Crab, imitation	1
Gefilte Fish, in jellied broth	3
Gefilte Fish, sweet w/broth	2
Grouper	1
Haddock, baked or broiled	1
Halibut	2
Herring, pickled	15
Lobster, boiled or steamed	1
Lox	4
Lox, imitation	2
Mackerel, baked or broiled	15
Mussels, boiled or steamed	4
Ocean Perch	2
Oyster, boiled or steamed	4

fat (grams): 0 5 10 15 20 25

* Counts are based on 3-ounce servings. Canned seafood items are assumed to be drained.

57

SEAFOOD*, Part 2

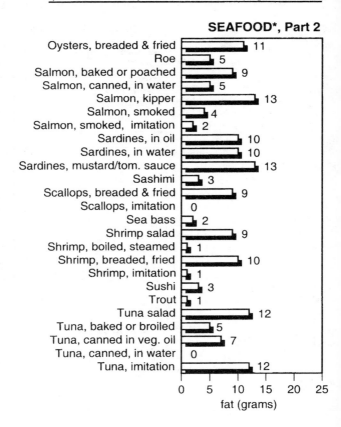

	fat (grams)
Oysters, breaded & fried	11
Roe	5
Salmon, baked or poached	9
Salmon, canned, in water	5
Salmon, kipper	13
Salmon, smoked	4
Salmon, smoked, imitation	2
Sardines, in oil	10
Sardines, in water	10
Sardines, mustard/tom. sauce	13
Sashimi	3
Scallops, breaded & fried	9
Scallops, imitation	0
Sea bass	2
Shrimp salad	9
Shrimp, boiled, steamed	1
Shrimp, breaded, fried	10
Shrimp, imitation	1
Sushi	3
Trout	1
Tuna salad	12
Tuna, baked or broiled	5
Tuna, canned in veg. oil	7
Tuna, canned, in water	0
Tuna, imitation	12

* Counts are based on 3-ounce servings. Canned seafood
items are assumed to be drained.

SNACKS AND CHIPS: Part 1*

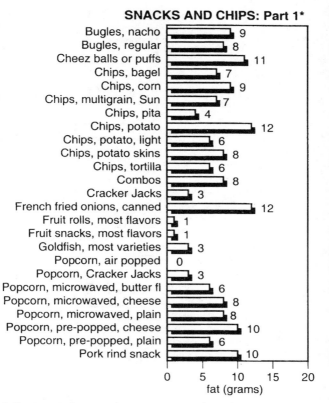

Snack	fat (grams)
Bugles, nacho	9
Bugles, regular	8
Cheez balls or puffs	11
Chips, bagel	7
Chips, corn	9
Chips, multigrain, Sun	7
Chips, pita	4
Chips, potato	12
Chips, potato, light	6
Chips, potato skins	8
Chips, tortilla	6
Combos	8
Cracker Jacks	3
French fried onions, canned	12
Fruit rolls, most flavors	1
Fruit snacks, most flavors	1
Goldfish, most varieties	3
Popcorn, air popped	0
Popcorn, Cracker Jacks	3
Popcorn, microwaved, butter fl	6
Popcorn, microwaved, cheese	8
Popcorn, microwaved, plain	8
Popcorn, pre-popped, cheese	10
Popcorn, pre-popped, plain	6
Pork rind snack	10

* For ease of comparison, counts are based on one-ounce
servings. For popcorn, 1 ounce unpopped = 2 cups popped.
Adjust count to reflect amount consumed.

SNACKS AND CHIPS: Part 2*

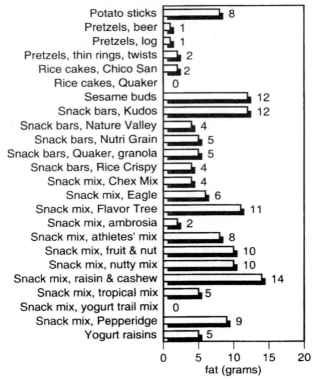

Snack	fat (grams)
Potato sticks	8
Pretzels, beer	1
Pretzels, log	1
Pretzels, thin rings, twists	2
Rice cakes, Chico San	2
Rice cakes, Quaker	0
Sesame buds	12
Snack bars, Kudos	12
Snack bars, Nature Valley	4
Snack bars, Nutri Grain	5
Snack bars, Quaker, granola	5
Snack bars, Rice Crispy	4
Snack mix, Chex Mix	4
Snack mix, Eagle	6
Snack mix, Flavor Tree	11
Snack mix, ambrosia	2
Snack mix, athletes' mix	8
Snack mix, fruit & nut	10
Snack mix, nutty mix	10
Snack mix, raisin & cashew	14
Snack mix, tropical mix	5
Snack mix, yogurt trail mix	0
Snack mix, Pepperidge	9
Yogurt raisins	5

fat (grams)

* For ease of comparison, counts are based on one-ounce
servings. For popcorn, 1 ounce unpopped = 2 cups popped.
Adjust count to reflect amount consumed.

SOUP*: Part 1

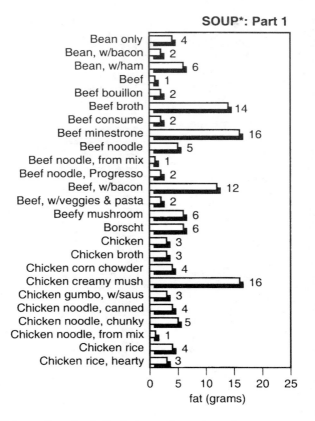

	fat (grams)
Bean only	4
Bean, w/bacon	2
Bean, w/ham	6
Beef	1
Beef bouillon	2
Beef broth	14
Beef consume	2
Beef minestrone	16
Beef noodle	5
Beef noodle, from mix	1
Beef noodle, Progresso	2
Beef, w/bacon	12
Beef, w/veggies & pasta	2
Beefy mushroom	6
Borscht	6
Chicken	3
Chicken broth	3
Chicken corn chowder	4
Chicken creamy mush	16
Chicken gumbo, w/saus	3
Chicken noodle, canned	4
Chicken noodle, chunky	5
Chicken noodle, from mix	1
Chicken rice	4
Chicken rice, hearty	3

* Unless otherwise indicated, counts are based on one-cup servings.

SOUP*, Part 2

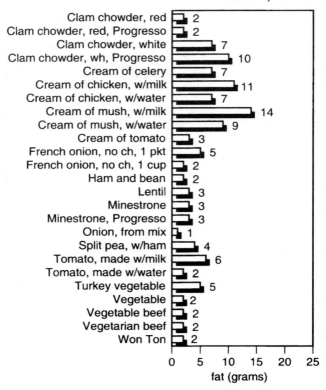

	fat (grams)
Clam chowder, red	2
Clam chowder, red, Progresso	2
Clam chowder, white	7
Clam chowder, wh, Progresso	10
Cream of celery	7
Cream of chicken, w/milk	11
Cream of chicken, w/water	7
Cream of mush, w/milk	14
Cream of mush, w/water	9
Cream of tomato	3
French onion, no ch, 1 pkt	5
French onion, no ch, 1 cup	2
Ham and bean	2
Lentil	3
Minestrone	3
Minestrone, Progresso	3
Onion, from mix	1
Split pea, w/ham	4
Tomato, made w/milk	6
Tomato, made w/water	2
Turkey vegetable	5
Vegetable	2
Vegetable beef	2
Vegetarian beef	2
Won Ton	2

* Unless otherwise indicated, counts are based on one-cup servings.

Sweets: CAKES*, Part 1

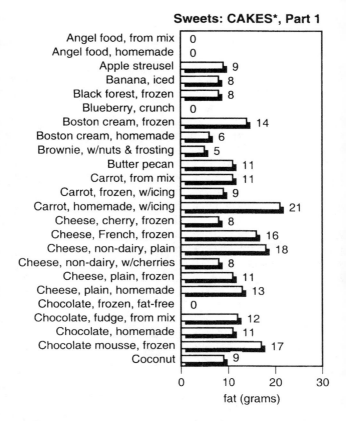

Food	fat (grams)
Angel food, from mix	0
Angel food, homemade	0
Apple streusel	9
Banana, iced	8
Black forest, frozen	8
Blueberry, crunch	0
Boston cream, frozen	14
Boston cream, homemade	6
Brownie, w/nuts & frosting	5
Butter pecan	11
Carrot, from mix	11
Carrot, frozen, w/icing	9
Carrot, homemade, w/icing	21
Cheese, cherry, frozen	8
Cheese, French, frozen	16
Cheese, non-dairy, plain	18
Cheese, non-dairy, w/cherries	8
Cheese, plain, frozen	11
Cheese, plain, homemade	13
Chocolate, frozen, fat-free	0
Chocolate, fudge, from mix	12
Chocolate, homemade	11
Chocolate mousse, frozen	17
Coconut	9

* Counts are based on average-size pieces and slices,
where appropriate, as indicated on package.

63

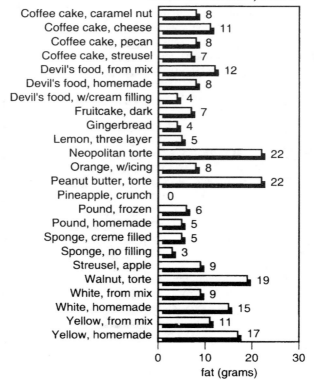

Sweets: CAKES*, Part 2

Cake	fat (grams)
Coffee cake, caramel nut	8
Coffee cake, cheese	11
Coffee cake, pecan	8
Coffee cake, streusel	7
Devil's food, from mix	12
Devil's food, homemade	8
Devil's food, w/cream filling	4
Fruitcake, dark	7
Gingerbread	4
Lemon, three layer	5
Neopolitan torte	22
Orange, w/icing	8
Peanut butter, torte	22
Pineapple, crunch	0
Pound, frozen	6
Pound, homemade	5
Sponge, creme filled	5
Sponge, no filling	3
Streusel, apple	9
Walnut, torte	19
White, from mix	9
White, homemade	15
Yellow, from mix	11
Yellow, homemade	17

fat (grams)

* Counts are based on average-size pieces and slices,
where appropriate, as indicated on package.

64

Sweets: SNACK CAKES*

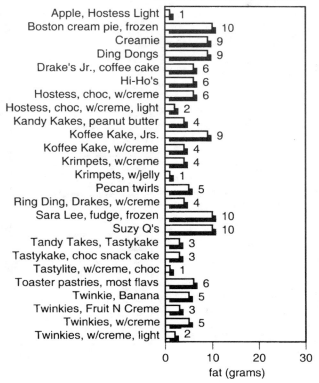

	fat (grams)
Apple, Hostess Light	1
Boston cream pie, frozen	10
Creamie	9
Ding Dongs	9
Drake's Jr., coffee cake	6
Hi-Ho's	6
Hostess, choc, w/creme	6
Hostess, choc, w/creme, light	2
Kandy Kakes, peanut butter	4
Koffee Kake, Jrs.	9
Koffee Kake, w/creme	4
Krimpets, w/creme	4
Krimpets, w/jelly	1
Pecan twirls	5
Ring Ding, Drakes, w/creme	4
Sara Lee, fudge, frozen	10
Suzy Q's	10
Tandy Takes, Tastykake	3
Tastykake, choc snack cake	3
Tastylite, w/creme, choc	1
Toaster pastries, most flavs	6
Twinkie, Banana	5
Twinkies, Fruit N Creme	3
Twinkies, w/creme	5
Twinkies, w/creme, light	2

* Counts are based on average-size pieces and slices,
  where appropriate, as indicated on package.

Sweets: CANDY*, Part 1

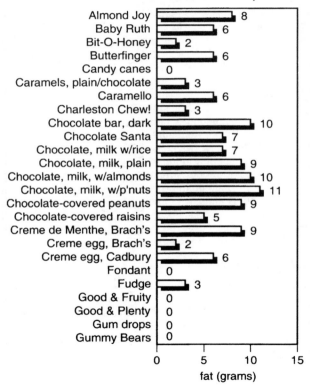

Candy	fat (grams)
Almond Joy	8
Baby Ruth	6
Bit-O-Honey	2
Butterfinger	6
Candy canes	0
Caramels, plain/chocolate	3
Caramello	6
Charleston Chew!	3
Chocolate bar, dark	10
Chocolate Santa	7
Chocolate, milk w/rice	7
Chocolate, milk, plain	9
Chocolate, milk, w/almonds	10
Chocolate, milk, w/p'nuts	11
Chocolate-covered peanuts	9
Chocolate-covered raisins	5
Creme de Menthe, Brach's	9
Creme egg, Brach's	2
Creme egg, Cadbury	6
Fondant	0
Fudge	3
Good & Fruity	0
Good & Plenty	0
Gum drops	0
Gummy Bears	0

fat (grams)

* For ease of comparison, counts are based on one-ounce
servings. Adjust counts to reflect quantities consumed.

Sweets: CANDY*, Part 2

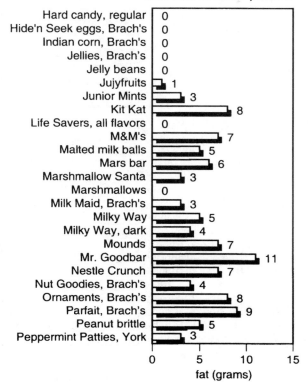

	fat (grams)
Hard candy, regular	0
Hide'n Seek eggs, Brach's	0
Indian corn, Brach's	0
Jellies, Brach's	0
Jelly beans	0
Jujyfruits	1
Junior Mints	3
Kit Kat	8
Life Savers, all flavors	0
M&M's	7
Malted milk balls	5
Mars bar	6
Marshmallow Santa	3
Marshmallows	0
Milk Maid, Brach's	3
Milky Way	5
Milky Way, dark	4
Mounds	7
Mr. Goodbar	11
Nestle Crunch	7
Nut Goodies, Brach's	4
Ornaments, Brach's	8
Parfait, Brach's	9
Peanut brittle	5
Peppermint Patties, York	3

fat (grams)

* For ease of comparison, counts are based on one-ounce
servings. Adjust counts to reflect quantities consumed.

Sweets: CANDY*, Part 3

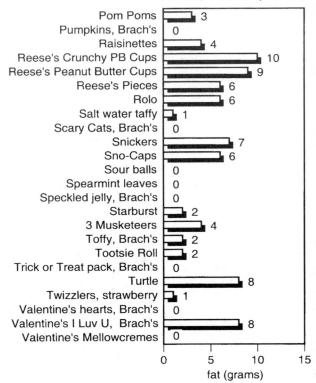

	fat (grams)
Pom Poms	3
Pumpkins, Brach's	0
Raisinettes	4
Reese's Crunchy PB Cups	10
Reese's Peanut Butter Cups	9
Reese's Pieces	6
Rolo	6
Salt water taffy	1
Scary Cats, Brach's	0
Snickers	7
Sno-Caps	6
Sour balls	0
Spearmint leaves	0
Speckled jelly, Brach's	0
Starburst	2
3 Musketeers	4
Toffy, Brach's	2
Tootsie Roll	2
Trick or Treat pack, Brach's	0
Turtle	8
Twizzlers, strawberry	1
Valentine's hearts, Brach's	0
Valentine's I Luv U, Brach's	8
Valentine's Mellowcremes	0

· * For ease of comparison, counts are based on one-ounce servings. Adjust counts to reflect quantities consumed.

Sweets: COOKIES*, Part 1

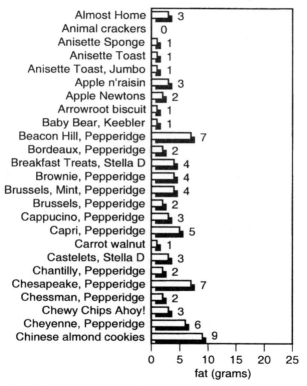

	fat (grams)
Almost Home	3
Animal crackers	0
Anisette Sponge	1
Anisette Toast	1
Anisette Toast, Jumbo	1
Apple n'raisin	3
Apple Newtons	2
Arrowroot biscuit	1
Baby Bear, Keebler	1
Beacon Hill, Pepperidge	7
Bordeaux, Pepperidge	2
Breakfast Treats, Stella D	4
Brownie, Pepperidge	4
Brussels, Mint, Pepperidge	4
Brussels, Pepperidge	2
Cappucino, Pepperidge	3
Capri, Pepperidge	5
Carrot walnut	1
Castelets, Stella D	3
Chantilly, Pepperidge	2
Chesapeake, Pepperidge	7
Chessman, Pepperidge	2
Chewy Chips Ahoy!	3
Cheyenne, Pepperidge	6
Chinese almond cookies	9

* NOTE: For ease of comparison, counts are based on
single cookie servings. When more than one cookie is
consumed, counts should be adjusted accordingly.

Sweets: COOKIES, Part 2

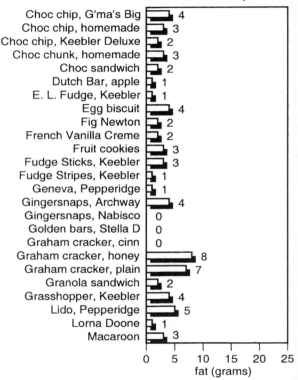

	fat (grams)
Choc chip, G'ma's Big	4
Choc chip, homemade	3
Choc chip, Keebler Deluxe	2
Choc chunk, homemade	3
Choc sandwich	2
Dutch Bar, apple	1
E. L. Fudge, Keebler	1
Egg biscuit	4
Fig Newton	2
French Vanilla Creme	2
Fruit cookies	3
Fudge Sticks, Keebler	3
Fudge Stripes, Keebler	1
Geneva, Pepperidge	1
Gingersnaps, Archway	4
Gingersnaps, Nabisco	0
Golden bars, Stella D	0
Graham cracker, cinn	0
Graham cracker, honey	8
Graham cracker, plain	7
Granola sandwich	2
Grasshopper, Keebler	4
Lido, Pepperidge	5
Lorna Doone	1
Macaroon	3

fat (grams) — 0 5 10 15 20 25

* NOTE: For ease of comparison, counts are based on
single cookie servings. When more than one cookie is
consumed, counts should be adjusted accordingly.

Sweets: COOKIES*, Part 3

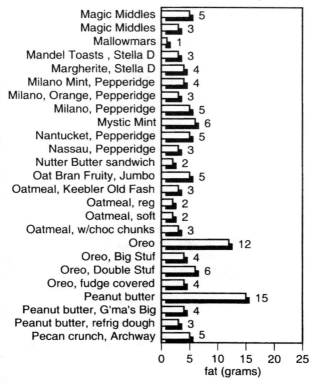

Cookie	fat (grams)
Magic Middles	5
Magic Middles	3
Mallowmars	1
Mandel Toasts , Stella D	3
Margherite, Stella D	4
Milano Mint, Pepperidge	4
Milano, Orange, Pepperidge	3
Milano, Pepperidge	5
Mystic Mint	6
Nantucket, Pepperidge	5
Nassau, Pepperidge	3
Nutter Butter sandwich	2
Oat Bran Fruity, Jumbo	5
Oatmeal, Keebler Old Fash	3
Oatmeal, reg	2
Oatmeal, soft	2
Oatmeal, w/choc chunks	3
Oreo	12
Oreo, Big Stuf	4
Oreo, Double Stuf	6
Oreo, fudge covered	4
Peanut butter	15
Peanut butter, G'ma's Big	4
Peanut butter, refrig dough	3
Pecan crunch, Archway	5

* NOTE: For ease of comparison, counts are based on
single cookie servings. When more than one cookie is
consumed, counts should be adjusted accordingly.

71

Alphabetical Chart
(for Hi-Low Comparison Charts, see pages 83 - 164)

Sweets: COOKIES*, Part 4

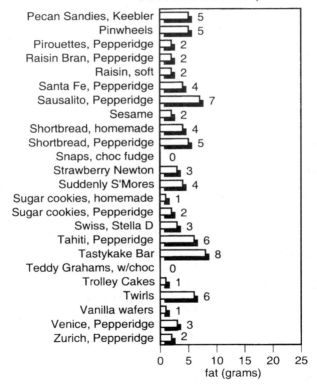

	fat (grams)
Pecan Sandies, Keebler	5
Pinwheels	5
Pirouettes, Pepperidge	2
Raisin Bran, Pepperidge	2
Raisin, soft	2
Santa Fe, Pepperidge	4
Sausalito, Pepperidge	7
Sesame	2
Shortbread, homemade	4
Shortbread, Pepperidge	5
Snaps, choc fudge	0
Strawberry Newton	3
Suddenly S'Mores	4
Sugar cookies, homemade	1
Sugar cookies, Pepperidge	2
Swiss, Stella D	3
Tahiti, Pepperidge	6
Tastykake Bar	8
Teddy Grahams, w/choc	0
Trolley Cakes	1
Twirls	6
Vanilla wafers	1
Venice, Pepperidge	3
Zurich, Pepperidge	2

* NOTE: For ease of comparison, counts are based on
single cookie servings. When more than one cookie is
consumed, counts should be adjusted accordingly.

Sweets: DONUTS*

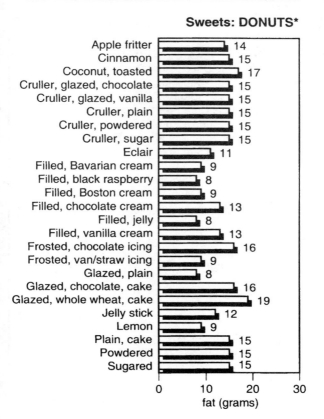

Donut	fat (grams)
Apple fritter	14
Cinnamon	15
Coconut, toasted	17
Cruller, glazed, chocolate	15
Cruller, glazed, vanilla	15
Cruller, plain	15
Cruller, powdered	15
Cruller, sugar	15
Eclair	11
Filled, Bavarian cream	9
Filled, black raspberry	8
Filled, Boston cream	9
Filled, chocolate cream	13
Filled, jelly	8
Filled, vanilla cream	13
Frosted, chocolate icing	16
Frosted, van/straw icing	9
Glazed, plain	8
Glazed, chocolate, cake	16
Glazed, whole wheat, cake	19
Jelly stick	12
Lemon	9
Plain, cake	15
Powdered	15
Sugared	15

fat (grams)

* Counts are based on average-size donuts.

Sweets: GUM & MINTS*

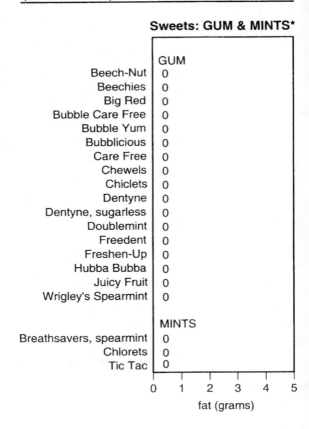

	GUM
Beech-Nut	0
Beechies	0
Big Red	0
Bubble Care Free	0
Bubble Yum	0
Bubblicious	0
Care Free	0
Chewels	0
Chiclets	0
Dentyne	0
Dentyne, sugarless	0
Doublemint	0
Freedent	0
Freshen-Up	0
Hubba Bubba	0
Juicy Fruit	0
Wrigley's Spearmint	0
	MINTS
Breathsavers, spearmint	0
Chlorets	0
Tic Tac	0

fat (grams)

* Counts are based on single sticks or mints.

Alphabetical Chart
(for Hi-Low Comparison Charts, see pages 83 - 164)

Sweets: ICE CREAM*

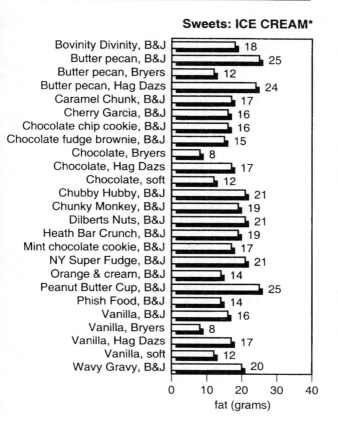

	fat (grams)
Bovinity Divinity, B&J	18
Butter pecan, B&J	25
Butter pecan, Bryers	12
Butter pecan, Hag Dazs	24
Caramel Chunk, B&J	17
Cherry Garcia, B&J	16
Chocolate chip cookie, B&J	16
Chocolate fudge brownie, B&J	15
Chocolate, Bryers	8
Chocolate, Hag Dazs	17
Chocolate, soft	12
Chubby Hubby, B&J	21
Chunky Monkey, B&J	19
Dilberts Nuts, B&J	21
Heath Bar Crunch, B&J	19
Mint chocolate cookie, B&J	17
NY Super Fudge, B&J	21
Orange & cream, B&J	14
Peanut Butter Cup, B&J	25
Phish Food, B&J	14
Vanilla, B&J	16
Vanilla, Bryers	8
Vanilla, Hag Dazs	17
Vanilla, soft	12
Wavy Gravy, B&J	20

* Counts are based on one-half cup servings. "B&J"
designates Ben & Jerry's brand.

Sweets: ICE CREAM CONES & BARS, ICE CREAM ALTERNATIVES AND PUDDINGS*

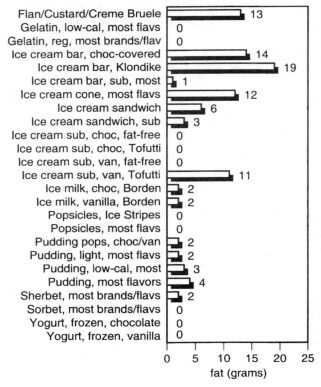

	fat (grams)
Flan/Custard/Creme Bruele	13
Gelatin, low-cal, most flavs	0
Gelatin, reg, most brands/flav	0
Ice cream bar, choc-covered	14
Ice cream bar, Klondike	19
Ice cream bar, sub, most	1
Ice cream cone, most flavs	12
Ice cream sandwich	6
Ice cream sandwich, sub	3
Ice cream sub, choc, fat-free	0
Ice cream sub, choc, Tofutti	0
Ice cream sub, van, fat-free	0
Ice cream sub, van, Tofutti	11
Ice milk, choc, Borden	2
Ice milk, vanilla, Borden	2
Popsicles, Ice Stripes	0
Popsicles, most flavs	0
Pudding pops, choc/van	2
Pudding, light, most flavs	2
Pudding, low-cal, most	3
Pudding, most flavors	4
Sherbet, most brands/flavs	2
Sorbet, most brands/flavs	0
Yogurt, frozen, chocolate	0
Yogurt, frozen, vanilla	0

* Counts are based on average- or one-half cup servings.
"Sub" designates non-dairy, ice cream substitute.

76

Sweets: PIES*

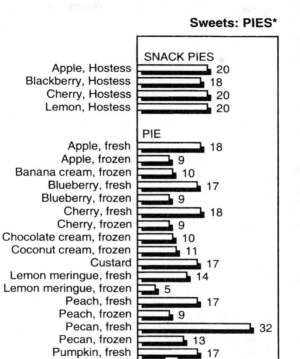

SNACK PIES	fat (grams)
Apple, Hostess	20
Blackberry, Hostess	18
Cherry, Hostess	20
Lemon, Hostess	20

PIE	fat (grams)
Apple, fresh	18
Apple, frozen	9
Banana cream, frozen	10
Blueberry, fresh	17
Blueberry, frozen	9
Cherry, fresh	18
Cherry, frozen	9
Chocolate cream, frozen	10
Coconut cream, frozen	11
Custard	17
Lemon meringue, fresh	14
Lemon meringue, frozen	5
Peach, fresh	17
Peach, frozen	9
Pecan, fresh	32
Pecan, frozen	13
Pumpkin, fresh	17
Pumpkin, frozen	6

0   10   20   30   40
fat (grams)

* Counts are based on average-size pieces and slices,
where appropriate, as indicated on package.

Sweets: SUGARS, SYRUPS, TOPPINGS AND JAMS*

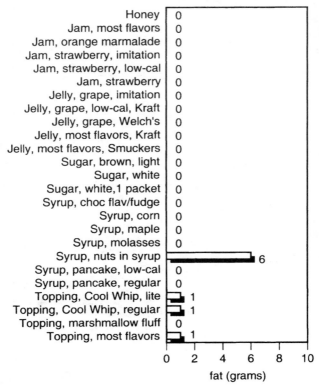

	fat (grams)
Honey	0
Jam, most flavors	0
Jam, orange marmalade	0
Jam, strawberry, imitation	0
Jam, strawberry, low-cal	0
Jam, strawberry	0
Jelly, grape, imitation	0
Jelly, grape, low-cal, Kraft	0
Jelly, grape, Welch's	0
Jelly, most flavors, Kraft	0
Jelly, most flavors, Smuckers	0
Sugar, brown, light	0
Sugar, white	0
Sugar, white, 1 packet	0
Syrup, choc flav/fudge	0
Syrup, corn	0
Syrup, maple	0
Syrup, molasses	0
Syrup, nuts in syrup	6
Syrup, pancake, low-cal	0
Syrup, pancake, regular	0
Topping, Cool Whip, lite	1
Topping, Cool Whip, regular	1
Topping, marshmallow fluff	0
Topping, most flavors	1

* Counts are based on single-tablespoon servings. Jams
and preserves can be assumed to have equal values.

VEGETABLES*, Part 1

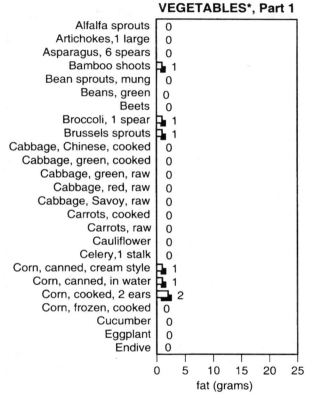

Vegetable	fat (grams)
Alfalfa sprouts	0
Artichokes, 1 large	0
Asparagus, 6 spears	0
Bamboo shoots	1
Bean sprouts, mung	0
Beans, green	0
Beets	0
Broccoli, 1 spear	1
Brussels sprouts	1
Cabbage, Chinese, cooked	0
Cabbage, green, cooked	0
Cabbage, green, raw	0
Cabbage, red, raw	0
Cabbage, Savoy, raw	0
Carrots, cooked	0
Carrots, raw	0
Cauliflower	0
Celery, 1 stalk	0
Corn, canned, cream style	1
Corn, canned, in water	1
Corn, cooked, 2 ears	2
Corn, frozen, cooked	0
Cucumber	0
Eggplant	0
Endive	0

* Unless otherwise indicated, counts are based on one-cup
servings. For vegetable juices, see the Fruits & Juices
section.

VEGETABLES*, Part 2

Vegetable	fat (grams)
Greens	1
Kale	1
Kohlrabi, stems	0
Lettuce, Boston, 1/4 head	0
Lettuce, Cos,1/4 head	0
Lettuce, Iceberg, 1/4 head	0
Lettuce, Romaine, 1/4 head	0
Mung bean, sprouted	0
Mushrooms, boiled/canned	1
Mushrooms, raw	0
Okra pods, 3 pods	0
Onions , cooked	0
Onions , raw	0
Parsnips	0
Pea pods, Chinese, cooked	0
Peas, green	1
Peppers, green, raw	0
Peppers, hot chili, 6	0
Peppers, red, raw	0
Plantain, cooked & sliced	0
Potato , au gratin	15
Potato salad	21
Potato, baked,1 medium	0
Potato, french fries, baked,14	6
Potato, french fries, 14	11

fat (grams)

* Unless otherwise indicated, counts are based on one-cup
servings. For vegetable juices, see the Fruits & Juices
section.

80

VEGETABLES*, Part 3

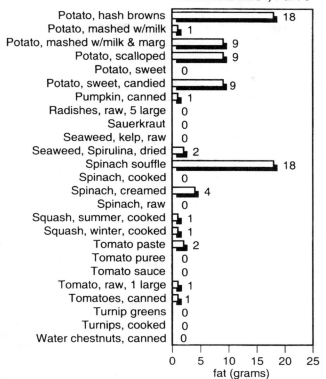

	fat (grams)
Potato, hash browns	18
Potato, mashed w/milk	1
Potato, mashed w/milk & marg	9
Potato, scalloped	9
Potato, sweet	0
Potato, sweet, candied	9
Pumpkin, canned	1
Radishes, raw, 5 large	0
Sauerkraut	0
Seaweed, kelp, raw	0
Seaweed, Spirulina, dried	2
Spinach souffle	18
Spinach, cooked	0
Spinach, creamed	4
Spinach, raw	0
Squash, summer, cooked	1
Squash, winter, cooked	1
Tomato paste	2
Tomato puree	0
Tomato sauce	0
Tomato, raw, 1 large	1
Tomatoes, canned	1
Turnip greens	0
Turnips, cooked	0
Water chestnuts, canned	0

0   5   10   15   20   25
fat (grams)

* Unless otherwise indicated, counts are based on one-cup
  servings. For vegetable juices, see the Fruits & Juices
  section.

VEGETARIAN CHOICES*

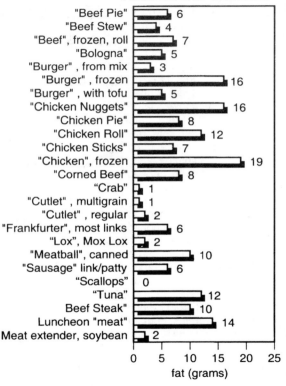

	fat (grams)
"Beef Pie"	6
"Beef Stew"	4
"Beef", frozen, roll	7
"Bologna"	5
"Burger" , from mix	3
"Burger" , frozen	16
"Burger" , with tofu	5
"Chicken Nuggets"	16
"Chicken Pie"	8
"Chicken Roll"	12
"Chicken Sticks"	7
"Chicken", frozen	19
"Corned Beef"	8
"Crab"	1
"Cutlet" , multigrain	1
"Cutlet" , regular	2
"Frankfurter", most links	6
"Lox", Mox Lox	2
"Meatball", canned	10
"Sausage" link/patty	6
"Scallops"	0
"Tuna"	12
Beef Steak"	10
Luncheon "meat"	14
Meat extender, soybean	2

0   5   10   15   20   25
fat (grams)

* Made from tofu, textured vegetable protein or a combination of both. Counts are based on 3-ounce servings.

HI-LOW COMPARISON CHARTS

BEVERAGES*, Part 1

	fat (grams)
Amaretto	0
Apple juice	0
Apricot cordial	0
Apricot nectar	0
Beer, dark	0
Beer, light	0
Beer, regular	0
Carrot juice	0
Champagne	0
Clam & tomato cocktail	0
Club soda	0
Coffee	0
Coffee-flavor grain bev	0
Cola, regular	0
Cola, sugar-free	0
Cranberry juice cocktail	0
Cranberry juice, sweetened	0
Creme de Cacao	0
Creme de Menthe	0
Crystal Light, most flavors	0
Fruit punch drink	0
Gin	0
Ginger ale, regular	0
Ginger ale, sugar-free	0
Grape drink	0

0   5   10   15   20   25
fat (grams)

* Counts for non-alcoholic drinks and beer are based on
8-fluid-ounce servings, for wine on 3 1/2-fluid-ounce
servings and, for hard liquor, on 1 1/2-fluid-ounce servings.

BEVERAGES*, Part 2

	fat (grams)
Grape juice	0
Grape soda	0
Grapefruit juice	0
Lemon-lime soda	0
Lemonade, from conc.	0
Limeade	0
Milk, nonfat	0
Milk, skim	0
Pineapple juice, unsweetened	0
Pineapple-grapefruit juice	0
Root beer, regular	0
Root beer, sugar-free	0
Rum	0
7 Up, regular	0
7 Up, sugar-free	0
Sprite, regular	0
Sprite, sugar-free	0
Tea	0
Tomato juice, 8 fl oz	0
Tonic water, regular	0
Tonic water, sugar-free	0
Vegetable juice cocktail	0
Vegetable juice, V-8	0
Vodka	0
Whisky	0

0   5   10   15   20   25
fat (grams)

* Counts for non-alcoholic drinks and beer are based on
8-fluid-ounce servings, for wine on 3 1/2-fluid-ounce
servings and, for hard liquor, on 1 1/2-fluid-ounce servings.

BEVERAGES*, Part 3

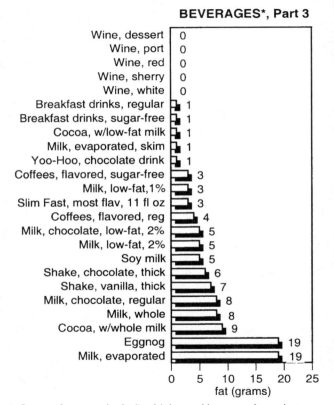

Beverage	fat (grams)
Wine, dessert	0
Wine, port	0
Wine, red	0
Wine, sherry	0
Wine, white	0
Breakfast drinks, regular	1
Breakfast drinks, sugar-free	1
Cocoa, w/low-fat milk	1
Milk, evaporated, skim	1
Yoo-Hoo, chocolate drink	1
Coffees, flavored, sugar-free	3
Milk, low-fat,1%	3
Slim Fast, most flav, 11 fl oz	3
Coffees, flavored, reg	4
Milk, chocolate, low-fat, 2%	5
Milk, low-fat, 2%	5
Soy milk	5
Shake, chocolate, thick	6
Shake, vanilla, thick	7
Milk, chocolate, regular	8
Milk, whole	8
Cocoa, w/whole milk	9
Eggnog	19
Milk, evaporated	19

fat (grams)

* Counts for non-alcoholic drinks and beer are based on
8-fluid-ounce servings, for wine on 3 1/2-fluid-ounce
servings and, for hard liquor, on 1 1/2-fluid-ounce servings.

86

Hi-Low Comparison Chart
(for Alphabetical Charts, see pages 1 - 82)

Bread, Crackers, Flours:
BAGELS*

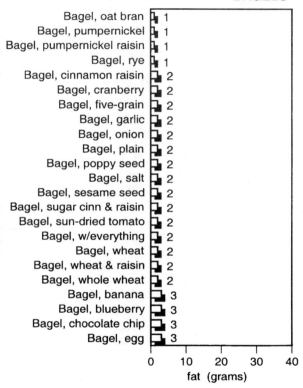

Bagel	fat (grams)
Bagel, oat bran	1
Bagel, pumpernickel	1
Bagel, pumpernickel raisin	1
Bagel, rye	1
Bagel, cinnamon raisin	2
Bagel, cranberry	2
Bagel, five-grain	2
Bagel, garlic	2
Bagel, onion	2
Bagel, plain	2
Bagel, poppy seed	2
Bagel, salt	2
Bagel, sesame seed	2
Bagel, sugar cinn & raisin	2
Bagel, sun-dried tomato	2
Bagel, w/everything	2
Bagel, wheat	2
Bagel, wheat & raisin	2
Bagel, whole wheat	2
Bagel, banana	3
Bagel, blueberry	3
Bagel, chocolate chip	3
Bagel, egg	3

fat (grams)

* Counts are based on one bagel, approximate weight:
3 ounces.

**Bread, Crackers, and Flour:
BISCUITS, ROLLS & MUFFINS***

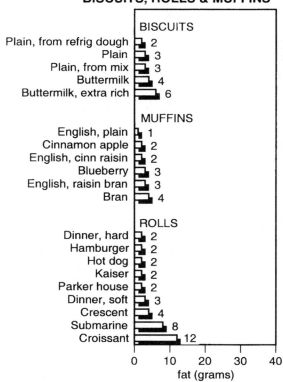

BISCUITS

Plain, from refrig dough	2
Plain	3
Plain, from mix	3
Buttermilk	4
Buttermilk, extra rich	6

MUFFINS

English, plain	1
Cinnamon apple	2
English, cinn raisin	2
Blueberry	3
English, raisin bran	3
Bran	4

ROLLS

Dinner, hard	2
Hamburger	2
Hot dog	2
Kaiser	2
Parker house	2
Dinner, soft	3
Crescent	4
Submarine	8
Croissant	12

0   10   20   30   40
fat (grams)

* Counts are based on single, average-size items. Average
sweet muffin is assumed to be 2 3/4 inches by 2 inches.
Average sweet and English muffin weight is 57 grams.

Bread, Crackers, and Flours:
BREAD*

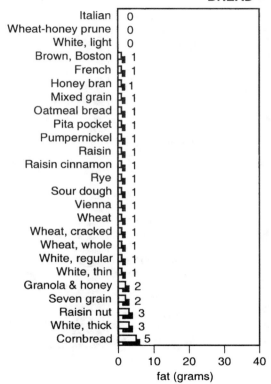

Bread	fat (grams)
Italian	0
Wheat-honey prune	0
White, light	0
Brown, Boston	1
French	1
Honey bran	1
Mixed grain	1
Oatmeal bread	1
Pita pocket	1
Pumpernickel	1
Raisin	1
Raisin cinnamon	1
Rye	1
Sour dough	1
Vienna	1
Wheat	1
Wheat, cracked	1
Wheat, whole	1
White, regular	1
White, thin	1
Granola & honey	2
Seven grain	2
Raisin nut	3
White, thick	3
Cornbread	5

* Counts are based on single, average-size slices.

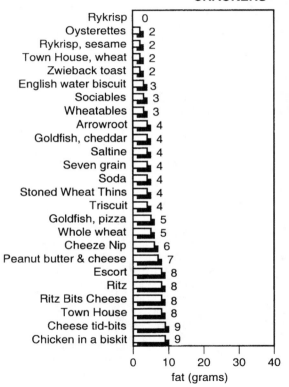

Hi-Low Comparison Chart
(for Alphabetical Charts, see pages 1 - 82)

Bread, Crackers, and Flours:
CRACKERS*

Cracker	fat (grams)
Rykrisp	0
Oysterettes	2
Rykrisp, sesame	2
Town House, wheat	2
Zwieback toast	2
English water biscuit	3
Sociables	3
Wheatables	3
Arrowroot	4
Goldfish, cheddar	4
Saltine	4
Seven grain	4
Soda	4
Stoned Wheat Thins	4
Triscuit	4
Goldfish, pizza	5
Whole wheat	5
Cheeze Nip	6
Peanut butter & cheese	7
Escort	8
Ritz	8
Ritz Bits Cheese	8
Town House	8
Cheese tid-bits	9
Chicken in a biskit	9

* For ease of comparison, counts are based on one-ounce
servings. Adjust counts to reflect quantities consumed.

90

Bread, Crackers, and Flours: DRY & CRISPY*

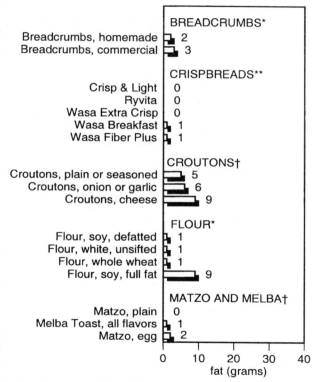

BREADCRUMBS*
Breadcrumbs, homemade 2
Breadcrumbs, commercial 3

CRISPBREADS**
Crisp & Light 0
Ryvita 0
Wasa Extra Crisp 0
Wasa Breakfast 1
Wasa Fiber Plus 1

CROUTONS†
Croutons, plain or seasoned 5
Croutons, onion or garlic 6
Croutons, cheese 9

FLOUR*
Flour, soy, defatted 1
Flour, white, unsifted 1
Flour, whole wheat 1
Flour, soy, full fat 9

MATZO AND MELBA†
Matzo, plain 0
Melba Toast, all flavors 1
Matzo, egg 2

0   10   20   30   40
fat (grams)

* Counts are based on 1/2- cup servings.

** Counts are based on single item.

† Counts are based on single-ounce servings.

Bread, Crackers, and Flours:
PANCAKES, STUFFING & MORE*

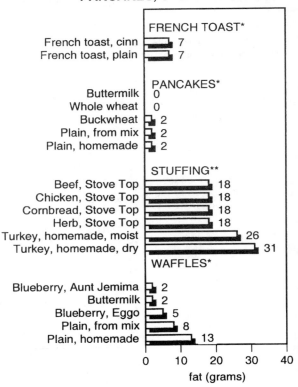

FRENCH TOAST*

French toast, cinn — 7
French toast, plain — 7

PANCAKES*

Buttermilk — 0
Whole wheat — 0
Buckwheat — 2
Plain, from mix — 2
Plain, homemade — 2

STUFFING**

Beef, Stove Top — 18
Chicken, Stove Top — 18
Cornbread, Stove Top — 18
Herb, Stove Top — 18
Turkey, homemade, moist — 26
Turkey, homemade, dry — 31

WAFFLES*

Blueberry, Aunt Jemima — 2
Buttermilk — 2
Blueberry, Eggo — 5
Plain, from mix — 8
Plain, homemade — 13

0   10   20   30   40
fat (grams)

* Counts are based on single slice, pancake, or waffle.
** Counts are based on 1/2-cup servings, prepared.

Hi-Low Comparison Chart
(for Alphabetical Charts, see pages 1 - 82)

CEREALS*, Part 1

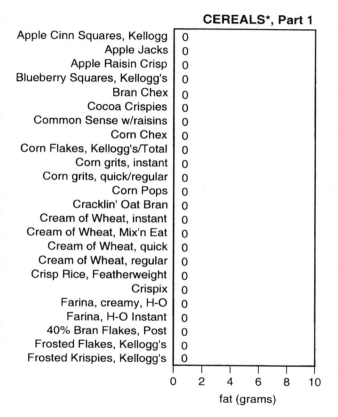

	fat (grams)
Apple Cinn Squares, Kellogg	0
Apple Jacks	0
Apple Raisin Crisp	0
Blueberry Squares, Kellogg's	0
Bran Chex	0
Cocoa Crispies	0
Common Sense w/raisins	0
Corn Chex	0
Corn Flakes, Kellogg's/Total	0
Corn grits, instant	0
Corn grits, quick/regular	0
Corn Pops	0
Cracklin' Oat Bran	0
Cream of Wheat, instant	0
Cream of Wheat, Mix'n Eat	0
Cream of Wheat, quick	0
Cream of Wheat, regular	0
Crisp Rice, Featherweight	0
Crispix	0
Farina, creamy, H-O	0
Farina, H-O Instant	0
40% Bran Flakes, Post	0
Frosted Flakes, Kellogg's	0
Frosted Krispies, Kellogg's	0

0   2   4   6   8   10

fat (grams)

* Counts are based on average-size servings (as indicated
on package) and without added milk.

93

CEREALS*, Part 2

	fat (grams)
Fruit Lites, Health Valley	0
Fruitful Bran	0
Fruity Marshmallow, Krispies	0
Grape Nuts Flakes	0
Grape-Nuts	0
Health Valley Flakes	0
Hominy grits, instant	0
Hominy grits, quick/regular	0
Honeycomb	0
Malt-O-Meal	0
Nutri-Grain	0
Nutri-Grain w/raisins	0
Product 19	0
Puffed Rice	0
Puffed Wheat	0
Raisin Squares, Kellogg's	0
Rice Chex	0
Rice Krispies	0
Shredded Wheat, Nutri-Grain	0
Shredded Wheat, Quaker	0
Special K	0
Super Golden Crisps	0
Super Sugar Crisp	0
Toasties, Post	0
Trix	0

```
0    2    4    6    8    10
          fat (grams)
```

* Counts are based on average-size servings (as indicated
  on package) and without added milk.

CEREALS*, Part 3

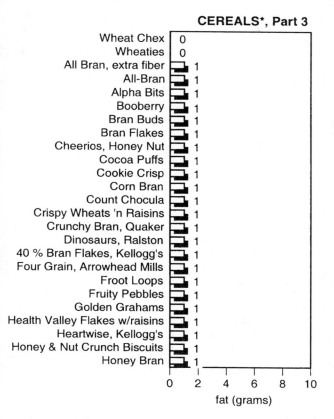

Cereal	fat (grams)
Wheat Chex	0
Wheaties	0
All Bran, extra fiber	1
All-Bran	1
Alpha Bits	1
Booberry	1
Bran Buds	1
Bran Flakes	1
Cheerios, Honey Nut	1
Cocoa Puffs	1
Cookie Crisp	1
Corn Bran	1
Count Chocula	1
Crispy Wheats 'n Raisins	1
Crunchy Bran, Quaker	1
Dinosaurs, Ralston	1
40 % Bran Flakes, Kellogg's	1
Four Grain, Arrowhead Mills	1
Froot Loops	1
Fruity Pebbles	1
Golden Grahams	1
Health Valley Flakes w/raisins	1
Heartwise, Kellogg's	1
Honey & Nut Crunch Biscuits	1
Honey Bran	1

fat (grams)

* Counts are based on average-size servings (as indicated
on package) and without added milk.

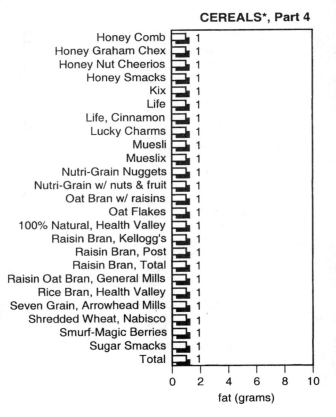

CEREALS*, Part 4

Cereal	fat (grams)
Honey Comb	1
Honey Graham Chex	1
Honey Nut Cheerios	1
Honey Smacks	1
Kix	1
Life	1
Life, Cinnamon	1
Lucky Charms	1
Muesli	1
Mueslix	1
Nutri-Grain Nuggets	1
Nutri-Grain w/ nuts & fruit	1
Oat Bran w/ raisins	1
Oat Flakes	1
100% Natural, Health Valley	1
Raisin Bran, Kellogg's	1
Raisin Bran, Post	1
Raisin Bran, Total	1
Raisin Oat Bran, General Mills	1
Rice Bran, Health Valley	1
Seven Grain, Arrowhead Mills	1
Shredded Wheat, Nabisco	1
Smurf-Magic Berries	1
Sugar Smacks	1
Total	1

fat (grams)

* Counts are based on average-size servings (as indicated
on package) and without added milk.

CEREALS*, Part 5

Cereal	fat (grams)
Wheat Flakes	1
Wheatena	1
Apple Cinnamon Cheerios	2
Cap'n Crunch's Crunchberries	2
Cheerios	2
Cheerios, Apple Cinnamon	2
Cinnamon Life	2
Cocoa Pebbles	2
Corn Flakes, Health Valley	2
Fruit & Fitness, Health Valley	2
Fruit and Fiber	2
Fruit Muesli, Ralston	2
Honey Bunches of Oats	2
Honey Graham Oh's	2
Muesli w/fruit	2
Oatmeal Crisp	2
Oatmeal, instant w/br sugar	2
Oatmeal, instant w/spice	2
Oatmeal, instant, flavored	2
Oatmeal, instant, H-O	2
Oatmeal, instant, plain	2
Oatmeal, quick, H-O	2
Oatmeal, regular	2
100% Bran	2

0 2 4 6 8 10
fat (grams)

* Counts are based on average-size servings (as indicated
on package) and without added milk.

CEREALS*, Part 6

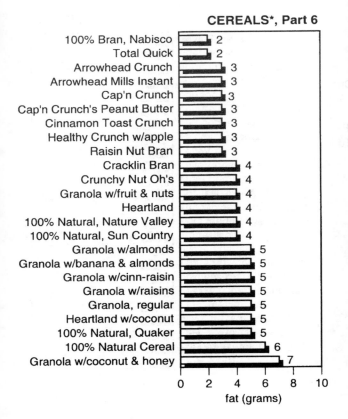

	fat (grams)
100% Bran, Nabisco	2
Total Quick	2
Arrowhead Crunch	3
Arrowhead Mills Instant	3
Cap'n Crunch	3
Cap'n Crunch's Peanut Butter	3
Cinnamon Toast Crunch	3
Healthy Crunch w/apple	3
Raisin Nut Bran	3
Cracklin Bran	4
Crunchy Nut Oh's	4
Granola w/fruit & nuts	4
Heartland	4
100% Natural, Nature Valley	4
100% Natural, Sun Country	4
Granola w/almonds	5
Granola w/banana & almonds	5
Granola w/cinn-raisin	5
Granola w/raisins	5
Granola, regular	5
Heartland w/coconut	5
100% Natural, Quaker	5
100% Natural Cereal	6
Granola w/coconut & honey	7

* Counts are based on average-size servings (as indicated
on package) and without added milk.

COMBINED AND FROZEN FOODS*,
Part 1

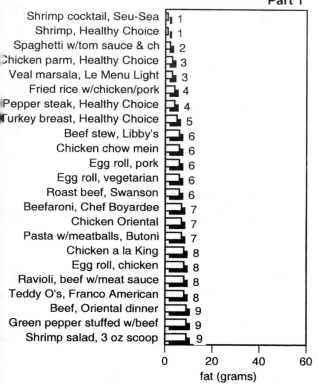

Food	fat (grams)
Shrimp cocktail, Seu-Sea	1
Shrimp, Healthy Choice	1
Spaghetti w/tom sauce & ch	2
Chicken parm, Healthy Choice	3
Veal marsala, Le Menu Light	3
Fried rice w/chicken/pork	4
Pepper steak, Healthy Choice	4
Turkey breast, Healthy Choice	5
Beef stew, Libby's	6
Chicken chow mein	6
Egg roll, pork	6
Egg roll, vegetarian	6
Roast beef, Swanson	6
Beefaroni, Chef Boyardee	7
Chicken Oriental	7
Pasta w/meatballs, Butoni	7
Chicken a la King	8
Egg roll, chicken	8
Ravioli, beef w/meat sauce	8
Teddy O's, Franco American	8
Beef, Oriental dinner	9
Green pepper stuffed w/beef	9
Shrimp salad, 3 oz scoop	9

fat (grams): 0   20   40   60

* Counts are based on average-size servings as indicated
on package. Adjust count to reflect amount consumed.

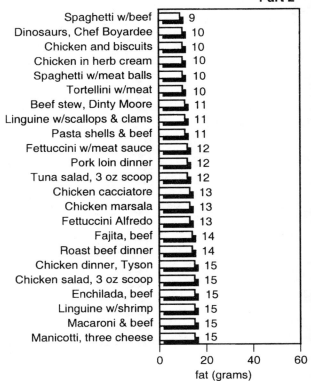

Hi-Low Comparison Chart
(for Alphabetical Charts, see pages 1 - 82)

COMBINED AND FROZEN FOODS*,
Part 2

Food	fat (grams)
Spaghetti w/beef	9
Dinosaurs, Chef Boyardee	10
Chicken and biscuits	10
Chicken in herb cream	10
Spaghetti w/meat balls	10
Tortellini w/meat	10
Beef stew, Dinty Moore	11
Linguine w/scallops & clams	11
Pasta shells & beef	11
Fettuccini w/meat sauce	12
Pork loin dinner	12
Tuna salad, 3 oz scoop	12
Chicken cacciatore	13
Chicken marsala	13
Fettuccini Alfredo	13
Fajita, beef	14
Roast beef dinner	14
Chicken dinner, Tyson	15
Chicken salad, 3 oz scoop	15
Enchilada, beef	15
Linguine w/shrimp	15
Macaroni & beef	15
Manicotti, three cheese	15

fat (grams) — 0   20   40   60

* Counts are based on average-size servings as indicated
on package. Adjust count to reflect amount consumed.

COMBINED AND FROZEN FOODS*,
Part 3

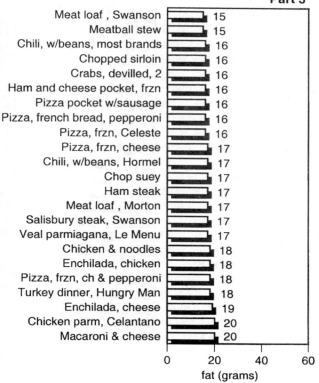

Food	fat (grams)
Meat loaf , Swanson	15
Meatball stew	15
Chili, w/beans, most brands	16
Chopped sirloin	16
Crabs, devilled, 2	16
Ham and cheese pocket, frzn	16
Pizza pocket w/sausage	16
Pizza, french bread, pepperoni	16
Pizza, frzn, Celeste	16
Pizza, frzn, cheese	17
Chili, w/beans, Hormel	17
Chop suey	17
Ham steak	17
Meat loaf , Morton	17
Salisbury steak, Swanson	17
Veal parmiagana, Le Menu	17
Chicken & noodles	18
Enchilada, chicken	18
Pizza, frzn, ch & pepperoni	18
Turkey dinner, Hungry Man	18
Enchilada, cheese	19
Chicken parm, Celantano	20
Macaroni & cheese	20

0   20   40   60
fat (grams)

* Counts are based on average-size servings as indicated
on package. Adjust count to reflect amount consumed.

COMBINED AND FROZEN FOODS*, Part 4

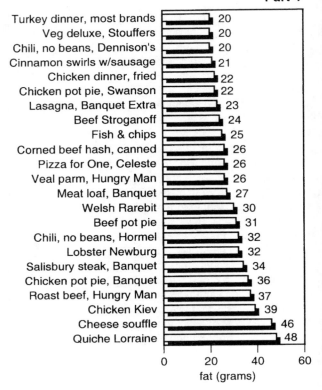

Food	fat (grams)
Turkey dinner, most brands	20
Veg deluxe, Stouffers	20
Chili, no beans, Dennison's	20
Cinnamon swirls w/sausage	21
Chicken dinner, fried	22
Chicken pot pie, Swanson	22
Lasagna, Banquet Extra	23
Beef Stroganoff	24
Fish & chips	25
Corned beef hash, canned	26
Pizza for One, Celeste	26
Veal parm, Hungry Man	26
Meat loaf, Banquet	27
Welsh Rarebit	30
Beef pot pie	31
Chili, no beans, Hormel	32
Lobster Newburg	32
Salisbury steak, Banquet	34
Chicken pot pie, Banquet	36
Roast beef, Hungry Man	37
Chicken Kiev	39
Cheese souffle	46
Quiche Lorraine	48

fat (grams) — 0 20 40 60

* Counts are based on average-size servings as indicated
on package. Adjust count to reflect amount consumed.

Dairy: CHEESE (HARD & SEMI-SOFT)*

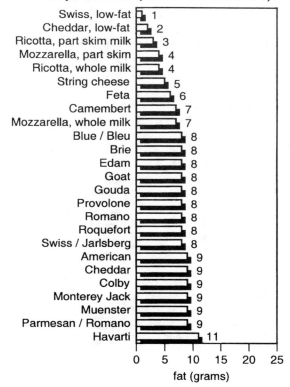

Cheese	fat (grams)
Swiss, low-fat	1
Cheddar, low-fat	2
Ricotta, part skim milk	3
Mozzarella, part skim	4
Ricotta, whole milk	4
String cheese	5
Feta	6
Camembert	7
Mozzarella, whole milk	7
Blue / Bleu	8
Brie	8
Edam	8
Goat	8
Gouda	8
Provolone	8
Romano	8
Roquefort	8
Swiss / Jarlsberg	8
American	9
Cheddar	9
Colby	9
Monterey Jack	9
Muenster	9
Parmesan / Romano	9
Havarti	11

0   5   10   15   20   25

fat (grams)

* Counts are based on one-ounce servings. Adjust count
to reflect amount consumed.

103

Dairy: CHEESES (SOFT),
CREAMS & SUBSTITUTES*

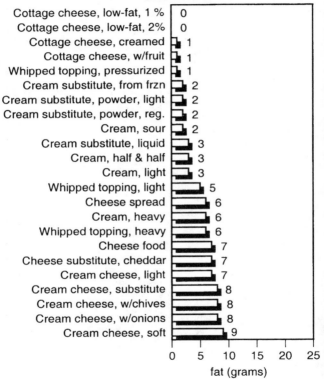

	fat (grams)
Cottage cheese, low-fat, 1 %	0
Cottage cheese, low-fat, 2%	0
Cottage cheese, creamed	1
Cottage cheese, w/fruit	1
Whipped topping, pressurized	1
Cream substitute, from frzn	2
Cream substitute, powder, light	2
Cream substitute, powder, reg.	2
Cream, sour	2
Cream substitute, liquid	3
Cream, half & half	3
Cream, light	3
Whipped topping, light	5
Cheese spread	6
Cream, heavy	6
Whipped topping, heavy	6
Cheese food	7
Cheese substitute, cheddar	7
Cream cheese, light	7
Cream cheese, substitute	8
Cream cheese, w/chives	8
Cream cheese, w/onions	8
Cream cheese, soft	9

* Counts are based on one-ounce servings of soft cheese
or one tablespoon of cream or whipped topping.

104

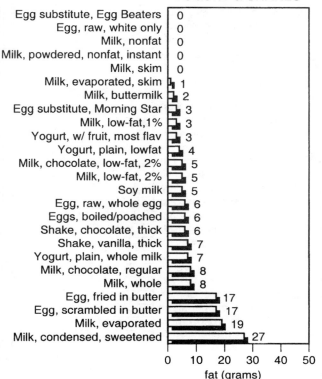

Hi-Low Comparison Chart
(for Alphabetical Charts, see pages 1 - 82)

Dairy: EGGS, MILK, YOGURT & SHAKES*

Food	fat (grams)
Egg substitute, Egg Beaters	0
Egg, raw, white only	0
Milk, nonfat	0
Milk, powdered, nonfat, instant	0
Milk, skim	0
Milk, evaporated, skim	1
Milk, buttermilk	2
Egg substitute, Morning Star	3
Milk, low-fat,1%	3
Yogurt, w/ fruit, most flav	3
Yogurt, plain, lowfat	4
Milk, chocolate, low-fat, 2%	5
Milk, low-fat, 2%	5
Soy milk	5
Egg, raw, whole egg	6
Eggs, boiled/poached	6
Shake, chocolate, thick	6
Shake, vanilla, thick	7
Yogurt, plain, whole milk	7
Milk, chocolate, regular	8
Milk, whole	8
Egg, fried in butter	17
Egg, scrambled in butter	17
Milk, evaporated	19
Milk, condensed, sweetened	27

fat (grams) — 0 10 20 30 40 50

* Counts based on one egg or equivalent egg substitute or 8 fluid ounces of milk, yogurt, or shake.

Dining Out: ASIAN*

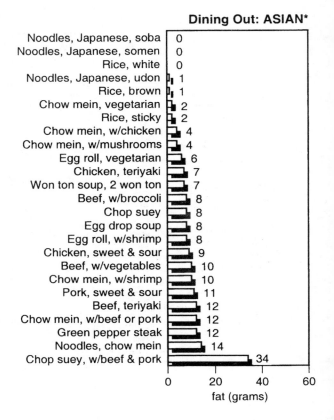

	fat (grams)
Noodles, Japanese, soba	0
Noodles, Japanese, somen	0
Rice, white	0
Noodles, Japanese, udon	1
Rice, brown	1
Chow mein, vegetarian	2
Rice, sticky	2
Chow mein, w/chicken	4
Chow mein, w/mushrooms	4
Egg roll, vegetarian	6
Chicken, teriyaki	7
Won ton soup, 2 won ton	7
Beef, w/broccoli	8
Chop suey	8
Egg drop soup	8
Egg roll, w/shrimp	8
Chicken, sweet & sour	9
Beef, w/vegetables	10
Chow mein, w/shrimp	10
Pork, sweet & sour	11
Beef, teriyaki	12
Chow mein, w/beef or pork	12
Green pepper steak	12
Noodles, chow mein	14
Chop suey, w/beef & pork	34

* Counts based on average-sized servings (for main dishes,
1 1/2 - 2 cups). Counts for main dishes include rice.

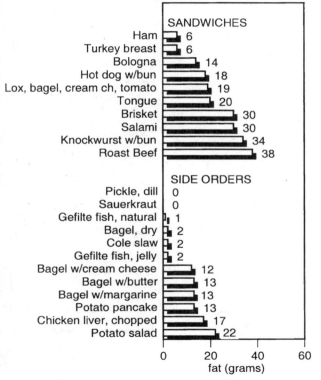

Dining Out: DELICATESSEN*

SANDWICHES

Ham	6
Turkey breast	6
Bologna	14
Hot dog w/bun	18
Lox, bagel, cream ch, tomato	19
Tongue	20
Brisket	30
Salami	30
Knockwurst w/bun	34
Roast Beef	38

SIDE ORDERS

Pickle, dill	0
Sauerkraut	0
Gefilte fish, natural	1
Bagel, dry	2
Cole slaw	2
Gefilte fish, jelly	2
Bagel w/cream cheese	12
Bagel w/butter	13
Bagel w/margarine	13
Potato pancake	13
Chicken liver, chopped	17
Potato salad	22

0   20   40   60
fat (grams)

* Unless otherwise indicated, counts based on average-size servings or sandwiches. Sandwich counts assume white or rye bread.

Dining Out: FRENCH AND
OTHER INTERNATIONAL DISHES*

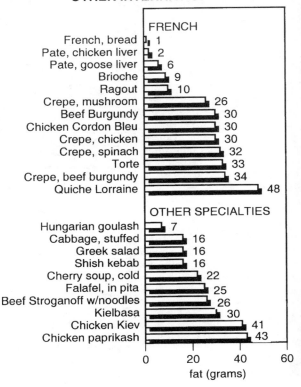

FRENCH

	fat (grams)
French, bread	1
Pate, chicken liver	2
Pate, goose liver	6
Brioche	9
Ragout	10
Crepe, mushroom	26
Beef Burgundy	30
Chicken Cordon Bleu	30
Crepe, chicken	30
Crepe, spinach	32
Torte	33
Crepe, beef burgundy	34
Quiche Lorraine	48

OTHER SPECIALTIES

	fat (grams)
Hungarian goulash	7
Cabbage, stuffed	16
Greek salad	16
Shish kebab	16
Cherry soup, cold	22
Falafel, in pita	25
Beef Stroganoff w/noodles	26
Kielbasa	30
Chicken Kiev	41
Chicken paprikash	43

fat (grams)

* Counts based on average-sized servings (for main dishes,
1 1/2 - 2 cups).

108

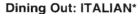

Hi-Low Comparison Chart
(for Alphabetical Charts, see pages 1 - 82)

Dining Out: ITALIAN*

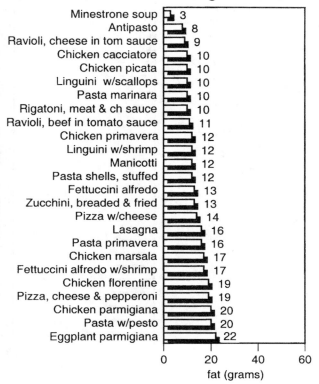

	fat (grams)
Minestrone soup	3
Antipasto	8
Ravioli, cheese in tom sauce	9
Chicken cacciatore	10
Chicken picata	10
Linguini w/scallops	10
Pasta marinara	10
Rigatoni, meat & ch sauce	10
Ravioli, beef in tomato sauce	11
Chicken primavera	12
Linguini w/shrimp	12
Manicotti	12
Pasta shells, stuffed	12
Fettuccini alfredo	13
Zucchini, breaded & fried	13
Pizza w/cheese	14
Lasagna	16
Pasta primavera	16
Chicken marsala	17
Fettuccini alfredo w/shrimp	17
Chicken florentine	19
Pizza, cheese & pepperoni	19
Chicken parmigiana	20
Pasta w/pesto	20
Eggplant parmigiana	22

fat (grams): 0 20 40 60

* Counts are based on average-sized servings (1 1/2 - 2 cups); for pizza, on 1/6 medium or 1/8 large pizza).

109

Dining Out: MEXICAN*

Food	fat (grams)
Picante sauce	0
Plantain, cooked	0
Tortilla, corn	1
Tortilla, wheat	2
Taco, shell	3
Tostada shell	4
Beans, refried	6
Churro	7
Burrito, beans	10
Enchilada, beef	10
Fajita, chicken	10
Fajita, steak	11
Taco, filling & sauce	11
Tostada w/sauce	11
Burrito, beef & beans	12
Enchilada, cheese	13
Enchilada, chicken	13
Taco salad w/salsa	15
Chili, w/beans	17
Burrito, beef	18
Nachos	18
Chimi	19
Enchirito w/sauce	20
Tamale dinner	20
Chili, no beans	29

fat (grams): 0   20   40   60

* Counts based on average-sized servings (for main dishes,
  1 1/2 - 2 cups).

110

Fast Food: ARBY'S*

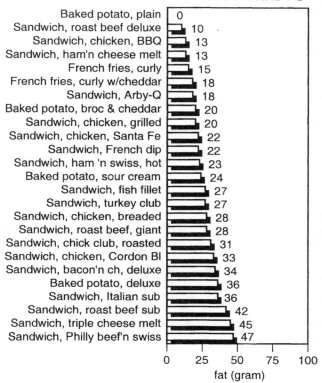

Item	fat (gram)
Baked potato, plain	0
Sandwich, roast beef deluxe	10
Sandwich, chicken, BBQ	13
Sandwich, ham'n cheese melt	13
French fries, curly	15
French fries, curly w/cheddar	18
Sandwich, Arby-Q	18
Baked potato, broc & cheddar	20
Sandwich, chicken, grilled	20
Sandwich, chicken, Santa Fe	22
Sandwich, French dip	22
Sandwich, ham 'n swiss, hot	23
Baked potato, sour cream	24
Sandwich, fish fillet	27
Sandwich, turkey club	27
Sandwich, chicken, breaded	28
Sandwich, roast beef, giant	28
Sandwich, chick club, roasted	31
Sandwich, chicken, Cordon Bl	33
Sandwich, bacon'n ch, deluxe	34
Baked potato, deluxe	36
Sandwich, Italian sub	36
Sandwich, roast beef sub	42
Sandwich, triple cheese melt	45
Sandwich, Philly beef'n swiss	47

fat (gram)

* Unless otherwise indicated, counts are based on average-
  size servings.

111

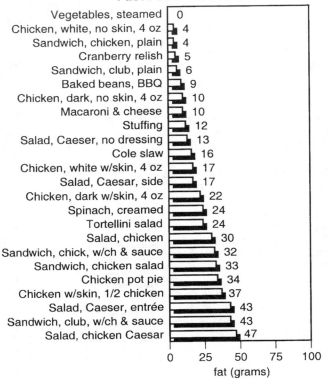

Hi-Low Comparison Chart
(for Alphabetical Charts, see pages 1 - 82)

Fast Food: BOSTON MARKET*

Food	fat (grams)
Vegetables, steamed	0
Chicken, white, no skin, 4 oz	4
Sandwich, chicken, plain	4
Cranberry relish	5
Sandwich, club, plain	6
Baked beans, BBQ	9
Chicken, dark, no skin, 4 oz	10
Macaroni & cheese	10
Stuffing	12
Salad, Caeser, no dressing	13
Cole slaw	16
Chicken, white w/skin, 4 oz	17
Salad, Caesar, side	17
Chicken, dark w/skin, 4 oz	22
Spinach, creamed	24
Tortellini salad	24
Salad, chicken	30
Sandwich, chick, w/ch & sauce	32
Sandwich, chicken salad	33
Chicken pot pie	34
Chicken w/skin, 1/2 chicken	37
Salad, Caeser, entrée	43
Sandwich, club, w/ch & sauce	43
Salad, chicken Caesar	47

fat (grams)

* Unless otherwise indicated, counts are based on average-size servings.

112

Hi-Low Comparison Chart
(for Alphabetical Charts, see pages 1 - 82)

Fast Food: BURGER KING*

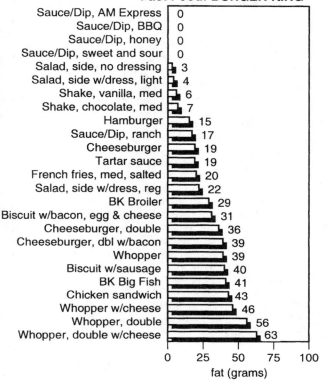

Item	fat (grams)
Sauce/Dip, AM Express	0
Sauce/Dip, BBQ	0
Sauce/Dip, honey	0
Sauce/Dip, sweet and sour	0
Salad, side, no dressing	3
Salad, side w/dress, light	4
Shake, vanilla, med	6
Shake, chocolate, med	7
Hamburger	15
Sauce/Dip, ranch	17
Cheeseburger	19
Tartar sauce	19
French fries, med, salted	20
Salad, side w/dress, reg	22
BK Broiler	29
Biscuit w/bacon, egg & cheese	31
Cheeseburger, double	36
Cheeseburger, dbl w/bacon	39
Whopper	39
Biscuit w/sausage	40
BK Big Fish	41
Chicken sandwich	43
Whopper w/cheese	46
Whopper, double	56
Whopper, double w/cheese	63

fat (grams)

* Unless otherwise indicated, counts are based on average-
size servings.

113

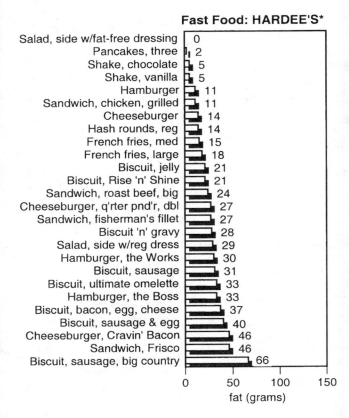

Hi-Low Comparison Chart
(for Alphabetical Charts, see pages 1 - 82)

Fast Food: HARDEE'S*

Item	fat (grams)
Salad, side w/fat-free dressing	0
Pancakes, three	2
Shake, chocolate	5
Shake, vanilla	5
Hamburger	11
Sandwich, chicken, grilled	11
Cheeseburger	14
Hash rounds, reg	14
French fries, med	15
French fries, large	18
Biscuit, jelly	21
Biscuit, Rise 'n' Shine	21
Sandwich, roast beef, big	24
Cheeseburger, q'rter pnd'r, dbl	27
Sandwich, fisherman's fillet	27
Biscuit 'n' gravy	28
Salad, side w/reg dress	29
Hamburger, the Works	30
Biscuit, sausage	31
Biscuit, ultimate omelette	33
Hamburger, the Boss	33
Biscuit, bacon, egg, cheese	37
Biscuit, sausage & egg	40
Cheeseburger, Cravin' Bacon	46
Sandwich, Frisco	46
Biscuit, sausage, big country	66

* Unless otherwise indicated, counts are based on average-size servings.

114

Fast Food: JACK IN THE BOX*

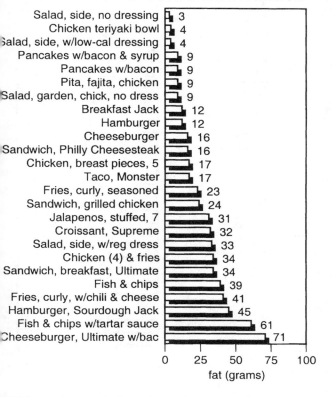

Item	fat (grams)
Salad, side, no dressing	3
Chicken teriyaki bowl	4
Salad, side, w/low-cal dressing	4
Pancakes w/bacon & syrup	9
Pancakes w/bacon	9
Pita, fajita, chicken	9
Salad, garden, chick, no dress	9
Breakfast Jack	12
Hamburger	12
Cheeseburger	16
Sandwich, Philly Cheesesteak	16
Chicken, breast pieces, 5	17
Taco, Monster	17
Fries, curly, seasoned	23
Sandwich, grilled chicken	24
Jalapenos, stuffed, 7	31
Croissant, Supreme	32
Salad, side, w/reg dress	33
Chicken (4) & fries	34
Sandwich, breakfast, Ultimate	34
Fish & chips	39
Fries, curly, w/chili & cheese	41
Hamburger, Sourdough Jack	45
Fish & chips w/tartar sauce	61
Cheeseburger, Ultimate w/bac	71

fat (grams)

* Unless otherwise indicated, counts are based on average-
size servings.

115

Fast Food: KFC*

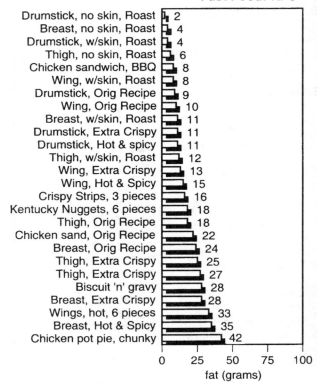

Item	fat (grams)
Drumstick, no skin, Roast	2
Breast, no skin, Roast	4
Drumstick, w/skin, Roast	4
Thigh, no skin, Roast	6
Chicken sandwich, BBQ	8
Wing, w/skin, Roast	8
Drumstick, Orig Recipe	9
Wing, Orig Recipe	10
Breast, w/skin, Roast	11
Drumstick, Extra Crispy	11
Drumstick, Hot & spicy	11
Thigh, w/skin, Roast	12
Wing, Extra Crispy	13
Wing, Hot & Spicy	15
Crispy Strips, 3 pieces	16
Kentucky Nuggets, 6 pieces	18
Thigh, Orig Recipe	18
Chicken sand, Orig Recipe	22
Breast, Orig Recipe	24
Thigh, Extra Crispy	25
Thigh, Extra Crispy	27
Biscuit 'n' gravy	28
Breast, Extra Crispy	28
Wings, hot, 6 pieces	33
Breast, Hot & Spicy	35
Chicken pot pie, chunky	42

fat (grams) — 0 25 50 75 100

* Unless otherwise indicated, counts are based on average-size servings.

116

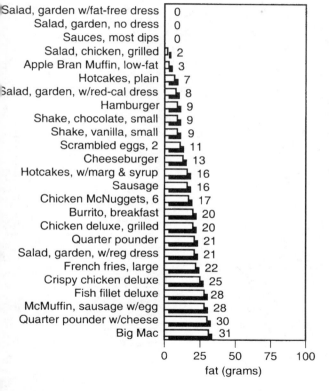

Hi-Low Comparison Chart
(for Alphabetical Charts, see pages 1 - 82)

Fast Food: MC DONALD'S*

Item	fat (grams)
Salad, garden w/fat-free dress	0
Salad, garden, no dress	0
Sauces, most dips	0
Salad, chicken, grilled	2
Apple Bran Muffin, low-fat	3
Hotcakes, plain	7
Salad, garden, w/red-cal dress	8
Hamburger	9
Shake, chocolate, small	9
Shake, vanilla, small	9
Scrambled eggs, 2	11
Cheeseburger	13
Hotcakes, w/marg & syrup	16
Sausage	16
Chicken McNuggets, 6	17
Burrito, breakfast	20
Chicken deluxe, grilled	20
Quarter pounder	21
Salad, garden, w/reg dress	21
French fries, large	22
Crispy chicken deluxe	25
Fish fillet deluxe	28
McMuffin, sausage w/egg	28
Quarter pounder w/cheese	30
Big Mac	31

0   25   50   75   100
fat (grams)

* Unless otherwise indicated, counts are based on average-size servings.

Hi-Low Comparison Chart
(for Alphabetical Charts, see pages 1 - 82)

Fast Food: PIZZA HUT*

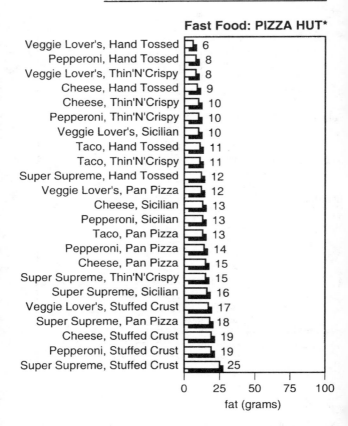

	fat (grams)
Veggie Lover's, Hand Tossed	6
Pepperoni, Hand Tossed	8
Veggie Lover's, Thin'N'Crispy	8
Cheese, Hand Tossed	9
Cheese, Thin'N'Crispy	10
Pepperoni, Thin'N'Crispy	10
Veggie Lover's, Sicilian	10
Taco, Hand Tossed	11
Taco, Thin'N'Crispy	11
Super Supreme, Hand Tossed	12
Veggie Lover's, Pan Pizza	12
Cheese, Sicilian	13
Pepperoni, Sicilian	13
Taco, Pan Pizza	13
Pepperoni, Pan Pizza	14
Cheese, Pan Pizza	15
Super Supreme, Thin'N'Crispy	15
Super Supreme, Sicilian	16
Veggie Lover's, Stuffed Crust	17
Super Supreme, Pan Pizza	18
Cheese, Stuffed Crust	19
Pepperoni, Stuffed Crust	19
Super Supreme, Stuffed Crust	25

0   25   50   75   100

fat (grams)

* Unless otherwise indicated, counts are based on average-size servings.

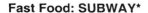

Hi-Low Comparison Chart
(for Alphabetical Charts, see pages 1 - 82)

Fast Food: SUBWAY*

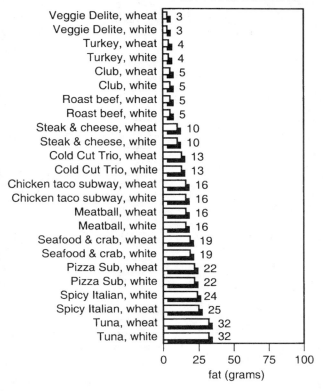

	fat (grams)
Veggie Delite, wheat	3
Veggie Delite, white	3
Turkey, wheat	4
Turkey, white	4
Club, wheat	5
Club, white	5
Roast beef, wheat	5
Roast beef, white	5
Steak & cheese, wheat	10
Steak & cheese, white	10
Cold Cut Trio, wheat	13
Cold Cut Trio, white	13
Chicken taco subway, wheat	16
Chicken taco subway, white	16
Meatball, wheat	16
Meatball, white	16
Seafood & crab, wheat	19
Seafood & crab, white	19
Pizza Sub, wheat	22
Pizza Sub, white	22
Spicy Italian, white	24
Spicy Italian, wheat	25
Tuna, wheat	32
Tuna, white	32

* Unless otherwise indicated, counts are based on average-
size servings.

119

Fast Food: TACO BELL*

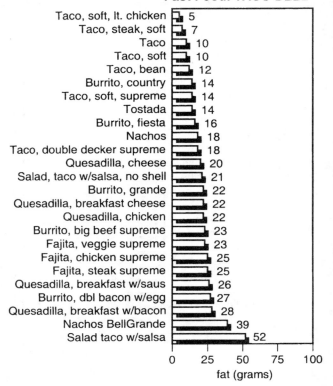

	fat (grams)
Taco, soft, lt. chicken	5
Taco, steak, soft	7
Taco	10
Taco, soft	10
Taco, bean	12
Burrito, country	14
Taco, soft, supreme	14
Tostada	14
Burrito, fiesta	16
Nachos	18
Taco, double decker supreme	18
Quesadilla, cheese	20
Salad, taco w/salsa, no shell	21
Burrito, grande	22
Quesadilla, breakfast cheese	22
Quesadilla, chicken	22
Burrito, big beef supreme	23
Fajita, veggie supreme	23
Fajita, chicken supreme	25
Fajita, steak supreme	25
Quesadilla, breakfast w/saus	26
Burrito, dbl bacon w/egg	27
Quesadilla, breakfast w/bacon	28
Nachos BellGrande	39
Salad taco w/salsa	52

* Unless otherwise indicated, counts are based on average-size servings.

Fast Food: WENDY'S*

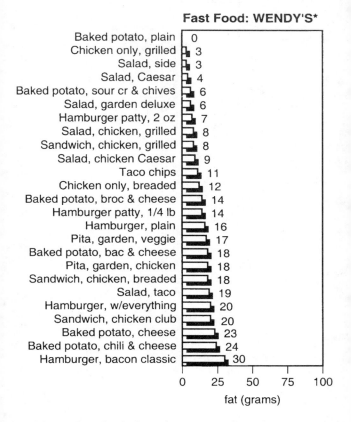

Item	fat (grams)
Baked potato, plain	0
Chicken only, grilled	3
Salad, side	3
Salad, Caesar	4
Baked potato, sour cr & chives	6
Salad, garden deluxe	6
Hamburger patty, 2 oz	7
Salad, chicken, grilled	8
Sandwich, chicken, grilled	8
Salad, chicken Caesar	9
Taco chips	11
Chicken only, breaded	12
Baked potato, broc & cheese	14
Hamburger patty, 1/4 lb	14
Hamburger, plain	16
Pita, garden, veggie	17
Baked potato, bac & cheese	18
Pita, garden, chicken	18
Sandwich, chicken, breaded	18
Salad, taco	19
Hamburger, w/everything	20
Sandwich, chicken club	20
Baked potato, cheese	23
Baked potato, chili & cheese	24
Hamburger, bacon classic	30

* Unless otherwise indicated, counts are based on average-size servings.

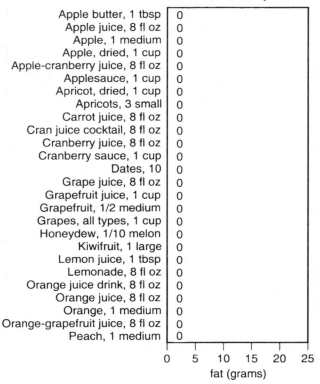

Hi-Low Comparison Chart
(for Alphabetical Charts, see pages 1 - 82)

**Fruits: FRESH & DRIED FRUITS
AND JUICES *, Part 1**

	fat (grams)
Apple butter, 1 tbsp	0
Apple juice, 8 fl oz	0
Apple, 1 medium	0
Apple, dried, 1 cup	0
Apple-cranberry juice, 8 fl oz	0
Applesauce, 1 cup	0
Apricot, dried, 1 cup	0
Apricots, 3 small	0
Carrot juice, 8 fl oz	0
Cran juice cocktail, 8 fl oz	0
Cranberry juice, 8 fl oz	0
Cranberry sauce, 1 cup	0
Dates, 10	0
Grape juice, 8 fl oz	0
Grapefruit juice, 1 cup	0
Grapefruit, 1/2 medium	0
Grapes, all types, 1 cup	0
Honeydew, 1/10 melon	0
Kiwifruit, 1 large	0
Lemon juice, 1 tbsp	0
Lemonade, 8 fl oz	0
Orange juice drink, 8 fl oz	0
Orange juice, 8 fl oz	0
Orange, 1 medium	0
Orange-grapefruit juice, 8 fl oz	0
Peach, 1 medium	0

0   5   10   15   20   25

fat (grams)

* Unless otherwise indicated, counts are based on whole,
fresh fruits.

122

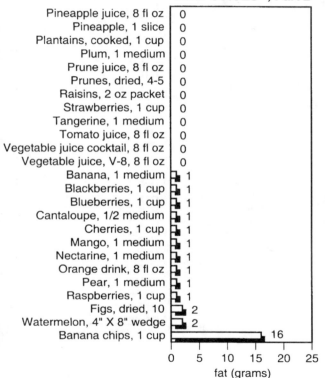

Hi-Low Comparison Chart
(for Alphabetical Charts, see pages 1 - 82)

Fruits: FRESH & DRIED FRUITS AND JUICES *, Part 2

Pineapple juice, 8 fl oz	0
Pineapple, 1 slice	0
Plantains, cooked, 1 cup	0
Plum, 1 medium	0
Prune juice, 8 fl oz	0
Prunes, dried, 4-5	0
Raisins, 2 oz packet	0
Strawberries, 1 cup	0
Tangerine, 1 medium	0
Tomato juice, 8 fl oz	0
Vegetable juice cocktail, 8 fl oz	0
Vegetable juice, V-8, 8 fl oz	0
Banana, 1 medium	1
Blackberries, 1 cup	1
Blueberries, 1 cup	1
Cantaloupe, 1/2 medium	1
Cherries, 1 cup	1
Mango, 1 medium	1
Nectarine, 1 medium	1
Orange drink, 8 fl oz	1
Pear, 1 medium	1
Raspberries, 1 cup	1
Figs, dried, 10	2
Watermelon, 4" X 8" wedge	2
Banana chips, 1 cup	16

0   5   10   15   20   25
fat (grams)

* Unless otherwise indicated, counts are based on whole, fresh fruits.

123

GRAVIES, SAUCES & DIPS*

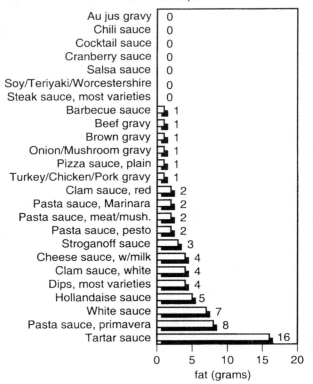

	fat (grams)
Au jus gravy	0
Chili sauce	0
Cocktail sauce	0
Cranberry sauce	0
Salsa sauce	0
Soy/Teriyaki/Worcestershire	0
Steak sauce, most varieties	0
Barbecue sauce	1
Beef gravy	1
Brown gravy	1
Onion/Mushroom gravy	1
Pizza sauce, plain	1
Turkey/Chicken/Pork gravy	1
Clam sauce, red	2
Pasta sauce, Marinara	2
Pasta sauce, meat/mush.	2
Pasta sauce, pesto	2
Stroganoff sauce	3
Cheese sauce, w/milk	4
Clam sauce, white	4
Dips, most varieties	4
Hollandaise sauce	5
White sauce	7
Pasta sauce, primavera	8
Tartar sauce	16

*Counts are based on one-quarter cup servings.

MEATS*, Part 1

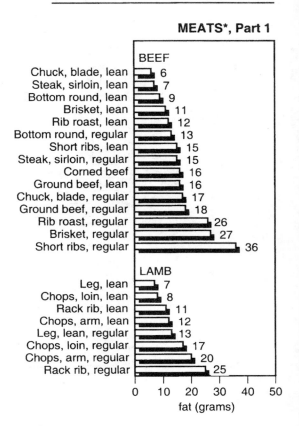

BEEF

	fat (grams)
Chuck, blade, lean	6
Steak, sirloin, lean	7
Bottom round, lean	9
Brisket, lean	11
Rib roast, lean	12
Bottom round, regular	13
Short ribs, lean	15
Steak, sirloin, regular	15
Corned beef	16
Ground beef, lean	16
Chuck, blade, regular	17
Ground beef, regular	18
Rib roast, regular	26
Brisket, regular	27
Short ribs, regular	36

LAMB

	fat (grams)
Leg, lean	7
Chops, loin, lean	8
Rack rib, lean	11
Chops, arm, lean	12
Leg, lean, regular	13
Chops, loin, regular	17
Chops, arm, regular	20
Rack rib, regular	25

fat (grams)

* Counts are based on 3-ounce servings.

125

MEATS*, Part 2

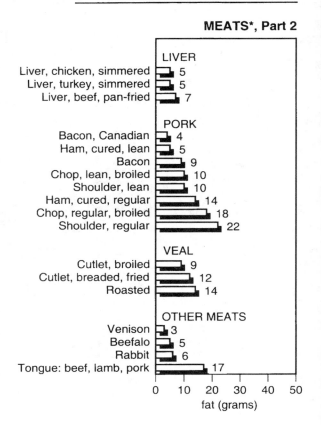

LIVER

Liver, chicken, simmered	5
Liver, turkey, simmered	5
Liver, beef, pan-fried	7

PORK

Bacon, Canadian	4
Ham, cured, lean	5
Bacon	9
Chop, lean, broiled	10
Shoulder, lean	10
Ham, cured, regular	14
Chop, regular, broiled	18
Shoulder, regular	22

VEAL

Cutlet, broiled	9
Cutlet, breaded, fried	12
Roasted	14

OTHER MEATS

Venison	3
Beefalo	5
Rabbit	6
Tongue: beef, lamb, pork	17

0   10   20   30   40   50
fat (grams)

* Counts are based on 3-ounce servings.

MEATS, PROCESSED*

Meat	fat (grams)
Chicken breast, sliced	2
Ham, lite/lean	2
Turkey breast/roll, lean, lite	2
Beef jerky	3
Corned beef, lite	3
Ham, boiled	3
Pastrami, turkey	3
Roast beef, lite/lean	3
Roast beef, regular	3
Turkey breast/roll, deli style	3
Bacon, Canadian	4
Chicken roll	4
Pastrami	4
Sausage, brown & serve, lean	5
Sausage, brown & serve	6
Bacon	9
Salami, turkey	12
Bologna	14
Corned beef	16
Hot dog	16
Salami, all beef	16
Sausage, Italian	17
Kielbasa, lite/lean	18
Kielbasa, regular	26
Salami, dry, hard	30

fat (grams) — 0 10 20 30 40

* Counts are based on 3-ounce servings.

127

Medications: COUGH DROPS & SYRUPS*

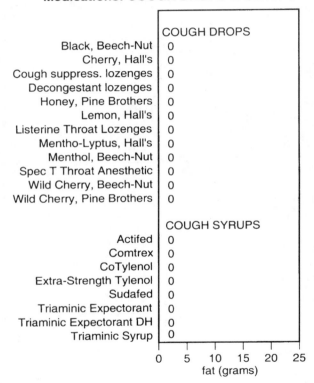

	COUGH DROPS
Black, Beech-Nut	0
Cherry, Hall's	0
Cough suppress. lozenges	0
Decongestant lozenges	0
Honey, Pine Brothers	0
Lemon, Hall's	0
Listerine Throat Lozenges	0
Mentho-Lyptus, Hall's	0
Menthol, Beech-Nut	0
Spec T Throat Anesthetic	0
Wild Cherry, Beech-Nut	0
Wild Cherry, Pine Brothers	0
	COUGH SYRUPS
Actifed	0
Comtrex	0
CoTylenol	0
Extra-Strength Tylenol	0
Sudafed	0
Triaminic Expectorant	0
Triaminic Expectorant DH	0
Triaminic Syrup	0

0   5   10   15   20   25
fat (grams)

* Counts are based on one cough drop or on recommended
doses for adults.

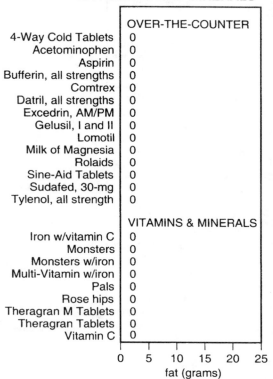

Hi-Low Comparison Chart
(for Alphabetical Charts, see pages 1 - 82)

Medications: OVER-THE-COUNTER REMEDIES & VITAMINS AND MINERALS*

	OVER-THE-COUNTER
4-Way Cold Tablets	0
Acetominophen	0
Aspirin	0
Bufferin, all strengths	0
Comtrex	0
Datril, all strengths	0
Excedrin, AM/PM	0
Gelusil, I and II	0
Lomotil	0
Milk of Magnesia	0
Rolaids	0
Sine-Aid Tablets	0
Sudafed, 30-mg	0
Tylenol, all strength	0
	VITAMINS & MINERALS
Iron w/vitamin C	0
Monsters	0
Monsters w/iron	0
Multi-Vitamin w/iron	0
Pals	0
Rose hips	0
Theragran M Tablets	0
Theragran Tablets	0
Vitamin C	0

0   5   10   15   20   25

fat (grams)

* Counts are based on recommended doses for adults.

MISCELLANEOUS FOODS*

	fat (grams)
Baking powder	0
Catsup	0
Chili powder	0
Cinnamon	0
Cocoa powder	0
Curry powder	0
Garlic powder	0
Gelatin, dry, 1 envelope	0
Ketchup	0
Mustard, w/ wine	0
Mustard, golden	0
Mustard, prepared yellow	0
Pepper, black	0
Pickles, dill, 1 medium	0
Pickles, fresh-pack, 2 slices	0
Pickles, sweet, 1 gherkin	0
Relish, sweet, chopped	0
Vinegar, balsamic	0
Vinegar, raspberry	0
Vinegar, red wine	0
Vinegar, white or cider	0
Yeast, 1 package	0
Olives, green, 3 medium	2
Olives, ripe, 3 medium	2
Chocolate, bitter baking	8

0   2   4   6   8   10
fat (grams)

* Unless otherwise indicated, counts are based on
a one-tablespoon serving.

130

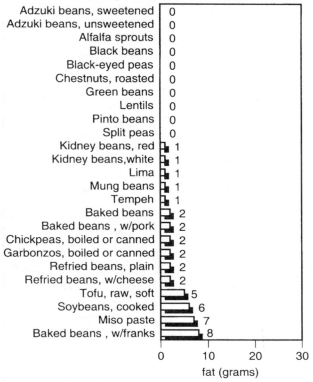

Hi-Low Comparison Chart
(for Alphabetical Charts, see pages 1 - 82)

NUTS, BEANS AND SEEDS*: Part 1

	fat (grams)
Adzuki beans, sweetened	0
Adzuki beans, unsweetened	0
Alfalfa sprouts	0
Black beans	0
Black-eyed peas	0
Chestnuts, roasted	0
Green beans	0
Lentils	0
Pinto beans	0
Split peas	0
Kidney beans, red	1
Kidney beans, white	1
Lima	1
Mung beans	1
Tempeh	1
Baked beans	2
Baked beans, w/pork	2
Chickpeas, boiled or canned	2
Garbonzos, boiled or canned	2
Refried beans, plain	2
Refried beans, w/cheese	2
Tofu, raw, soft	5
Soybeans, cooked	6
Miso paste	7
Baked beans, w/franks	8

* Unless otherwise indicated, counts are based on 1/2 cup tofu or cooked beans or one-ounce servings of raw nuts or seeds.

131

NUTS, BEANS AND SEEDS*: Part 2

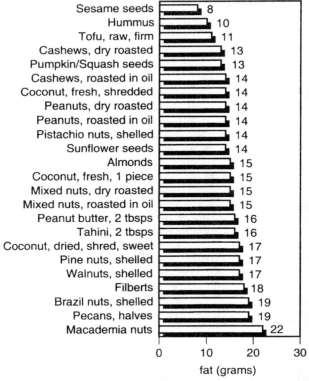

	fat (grams)
Sesame seeds	8
Hummus	10
Tofu, raw, firm	11
Cashews, dry roasted	13
Pumpkin/Squash seeds	13
Cashews, roasted in oil	14
Coconut, fresh, shredded	14
Peanuts, dry roasted	14
Peanuts, roasted in oil	14
Pistachio nuts, shelled	14
Sunflower seeds	14
Almonds	15
Coconut, fresh, 1 piece	15
Mixed nuts, dry roasted	15
Mixed nuts, roasted in oil	15
Peanut butter, 2 tbsps	16
Tahini, 2 tbsps	16
Coconut, dried, shred, sweet	17
Pine nuts, shelled	17
Walnuts, shelled	17
Filberts	18
Brazil nuts, shelled	19
Pecans, halves	19
Macadamia nuts	22

* Unless otherwise indicated, counts are based on 1/2 cup
tofu or cooked beans or one-ounce servings of raw nuts or
seeds.

OILS AND FATS*

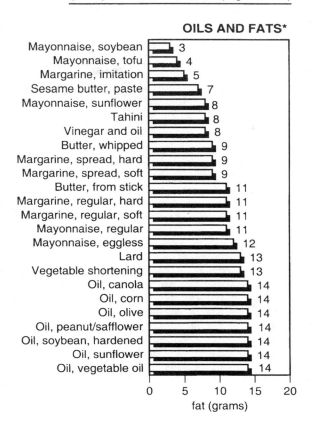

	fat (grams)
Mayonnaise, soybean	3
Mayonnaise, tofu	4
Margarine, imitation	5
Sesame butter, paste	7
Mayonnaise, sunflower	8
Tahini	8
Vinegar and oil	8
Butter, whipped	9
Margarine, spread, hard	9
Margarine, spread, soft	9
Butter, from stick	11
Margarine, regular, hard	11
Margarine, regular, soft	11
Mayonnaise, regular	11
Mayonnaise, eggless	12
Lard	13
Vegetable shortening	13
Oil, canola	14
Oil, corn	14
Oil, olive	14
Oil, peanut/safflower	14
Oil, soybean, hardened	14
Oil, sunflower	14
Oil, vegetable oil	14

0   5   10   15   20
fat (grams)

* Counts are based on 1-tablespoon servings.

133

PASTA, WHOLE GRAINS , RICE & NOODLES*, Part 1

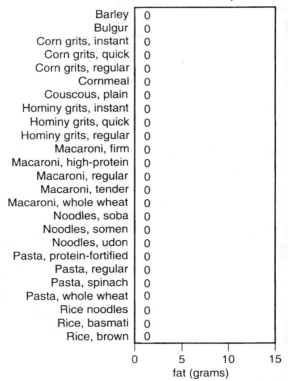

	fat (grams)
Barley	0
Bulgur	0
Corn grits, instant	0
Corn grits, quick	0
Corn grits, regular	0
Cornmeal	0
Couscous, plain	0
Hominy grits, instant	0
Hominy grits, quick	0
Hominy grits, regular	0
Macaroni, firm	0
Macaroni, high-protein	0
Macaroni, regular	0
Macaroni, tender	0
Macaroni, whole wheat	0
Noodles, soba	0
Noodles, somen	0
Noodles, udon	0
Pasta, protein-fortified	0
Pasta, regular	0
Pasta, spinach	0
Pasta, whole wheat	0
Rice noodles	0
Rice, basmati	0
Rice, brown	0

fat (grams)
0   5   10   15

* Counts are based on cooked, 1/2-cup servings.

PASTA, WHOLE GRAINS , RICE & NOODLES*, Part 2

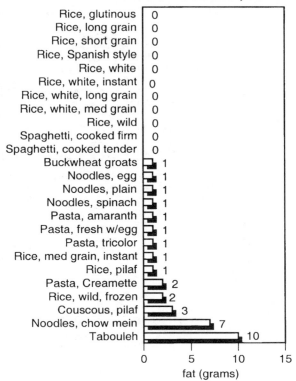

	fat (grams)
Rice, glutinous	0
Rice, long grain	0
Rice, short grain	0
Rice, Spanish style	0
Rice, white	0
Rice, white, instant	0
Rice, white, long grain	0
Rice, white, med grain	0
Rice, wild	0
Spaghetti, cooked firm	0
Spaghetti, cooked tender	0
Buckwheat groats	1
Noodles, egg	1
Noodles, plain	1
Noodles, spinach	1
Pasta, amaranth	1
Pasta, fresh w/egg	1
Pasta, tricolor	1
Rice, med grain, instant	1
Rice, pilaf	1
Pasta, Creamette	2
Rice, wild, frozen	2
Couscous, pilaf	3
Noodles, chow mein	7
Tabouleh	10

* Counts are based on cooked, 1/2-cup servings.

**Poultry: CHICKEN, TURKEY,
AND OTHER FOWL***

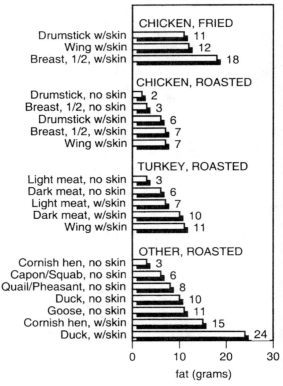

CHICKEN, FRIED

Drumstick w/skin	11
Wing w/skin	12
Breast, 1/2, w/skin	18

CHICKEN, ROASTED

Drumstick, no skin	2
Breast, 1/2, no skin	3
Drumstick w/skin	6
Breast, 1/2, w/skin	7
Wing w/skin	7

TURKEY, ROASTED

Light meat, no skin	3
Dark meat, no skin	6
Light meat, w/skin	7
Dark meat, w/skin	10
Wing w/skin	11

OTHER, ROASTED

Cornish hen, no skin	3
Capon/Squab, no skin	6
Quail/Pheasant, no skin	8
Duck, no skin	10
Goose, no skin	11
Cornish hen, w/skin	15
Duck, w/skin	24

0   10   20   30

fat (grams)

* Unless otherwise indicated, counts are based on 3-ounce
servings.

SALAD BAR CHOICES*

Salad Bar Choice	fat (grams)
Alfalfa sprouts	0
Bean sprouts	0
Beets	0
Broccoli	0
Cabbage	0
Cantaloupe/Honeydew	0
Carrots	0
Cauliflower	0
Croutons	0
Cucumber	0
Green pepper	0
Lettuce	0
Onions, chopped	0
Peaches	0
Peas	0
Chickpeas/Garbonzos	1
Cottage cheese	1
Gelatin parfait	2
Chinese noodles	3
Granola	3
Bacon bits	4
Pasta/Macaroni salad	5
Cheddar cheese	8
Egg, chopped	8
Sunflower seeds	14

fat (grams)

* Counts are based on one-quarter cup servings.

SALAD DRESSING*

Dressing	fat (grams)
Italian, low-cal	0
Mayonnaise, lowfat dress.	1
Russian/Thous Island, low-cal	1
Blue cheese, low-cal	2
Creamy Italian, low-cal	2
French, low-cal	2
Honey mustard	3
Vinaigrette, low-cal	3
Miracle Whip, light	4
Oil & vinegar dressing	4
Garlic, regular	5
Mayonnaise, light	5
Russian/Thous Island, reg	5
Blue cheese, reg	6
Creamy Italian, regular	6
Vinaigrette, regular	6
Miracle Whip, regular	7
Onion & chives	7
Caesar	8
Garlic, creamy	8
Oil & vinegar	8
Ranch	8
French, regular	9
Italian, regular	9
Mayonnaise, reg	11

0   5   10   15
fat (grams)

* For ease of comparison, counts are based on single
tablespoon servings. Adjust counts to reflect quantities
consumed.

SEAFOOD*, Part 1

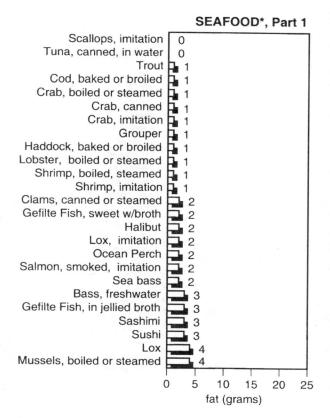

Food	fat (grams)
Scallops, imitation	0
Tuna, canned, in water	0
Trout	1
Cod, baked or broiled	1
Crab, boiled or steamed	1
Crab, canned	1
Crab, imitation	1
Grouper	1
Haddock, baked or broiled	1
Lobster, boiled or steamed	1
Shrimp, boiled, steamed	1
Shrimp, imitation	1
Clams, canned or steamed	2
Gefilte Fish, sweet w/broth	2
Halibut	2
Lox, imitation	2
Ocean Perch	2
Salmon, smoked, imitation	2
Sea bass	2
Bass, freshwater	3
Gefilte Fish, in jellied broth	3
Sashimi	3
Sushi	3
Lox	4
Mussels, boiled or steamed	4

* Counts are based on 3-ounce servings. Canned seafood
items are assumed to be drained.

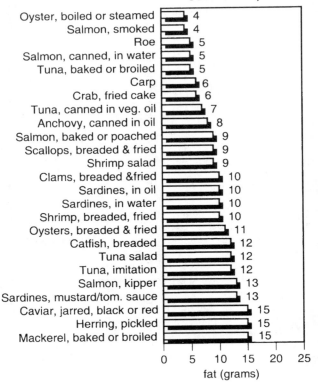

Hi-Low Comparison Chart
(for Alphabetical Charts, see pages 000-000)

SEAFOOD*, Part 2

Food	fat (grams)
Oyster, boiled or steamed	4
Salmon, smoked	4
Roe	5
Salmon, canned, in water	5
Tuna, baked or broiled	5
Carp	6
Crab, fried cake	6
Tuna, canned in veg. oil	7
Anchovy, canned in oil	8
Salmon, baked or poached	9
Scallops, breaded & fried	9
Shrimp salad	9
Clams, breaded &fried	10
Sardines, in oil	10
Sardines, in water	10
Shrimp, breaded, fried	10
Oysters, breaded & fried	11
Catfish, breaded	12
Tuna salad	12
Tuna, imitation	12
Salmon, kipper	13
Sardines, mustard/tom. sauce	13
Caviar, jarred, black or red	15
Herring, pickled	15
Mackerel, baked or broiled	15

0   5   10   15   20   25
fat (grams)

* Counts are based on 3-ounce servings. Canned seafood
items are assumed to be drained.

SNACKS: AND CHIPS: Part 1*

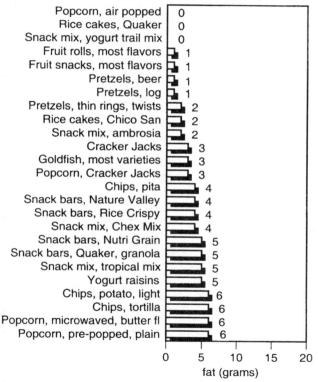

	fat (grams)
Popcorn, air popped	0
Rice cakes, Quaker	0
Snack mix, yogurt trail mix	0
Fruit rolls, most flavors	1
Fruit snacks, most flavors	1
Pretzels, beer	1
Pretzels, log	1
Pretzels, thin rings, twists	2
Rice cakes, Chico San	2
Snack mix, ambrosia	2
Cracker Jacks	3
Goldfish, most varieties	3
Popcorn, Cracker Jacks	3
Chips, pita	4
Snack bars, Nature Valley	4
Snack bars, Rice Crispy	4
Snack mix, Chex Mix	4
Snack bars, Nutri Grain	5
Snack bars, Quaker, granola	5
Snack mix, tropical mix	5
Yogurt raisins	5
Chips, potato, light	6
Chips, tortilla	6
Popcorn, microwaved, butter fl	6
Popcorn, pre-popped, plain	6

fat (grams) 0 5 10 15 20

* For ease of comparison, counts are based on one-ounce
servings. For popcorn, 1 ounce unpopped = 2 cups popped.
Adjust count to reflect amount consumed.

SNACKS AND CHIPS: Part 2*

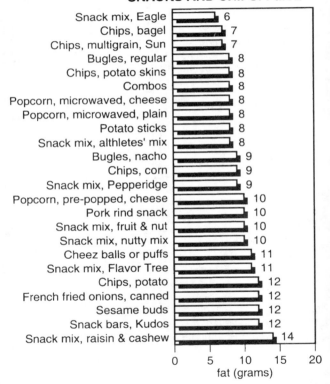

	fat (grams)
Snack mix, Eagle	6
Chips, bagel	7
Chips, multigrain, Sun	7
Bugles, regular	8
Chips, potato skins	8
Combos	8
Popcorn, microwaved, cheese	8
Popcorn, microwaved, plain	8
Potato sticks	8
Snack mix, althletes' mix	8
Bugles, nacho	9
Chips, corn	9
Snack mix, Pepperidge	9
Popcorn, pre-popped, cheese	10
Pork rind snack	10
Snack mix, fruit & nut	10
Snack mix, nutty mix	10
Cheez balls or puffs	11
Snack mix, Flavor Tree	11
Chips, potato	12
French fried onions, canned	12
Sesame buds	12
Snack bars, Kudos	12
Snack mix, raisin & cashew	14

fat (grams): 0 5 10 15 20

* For ease of comparison, counts are based on one-ounce
  servings. For popcorn, 1 ounce unpopped = 2 cups popped.
  Adjust count to reflect amount consumed.

SOUP*: Part 1

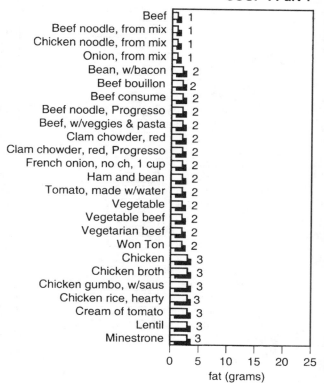

	fat (grams)
Beef	1
Beef noodle, from mix	1
Chicken noodle, from mix	1
Onion, from mix	1
Bean, w/bacon	2
Beef bouillon	2
Beef consume	2
Beef noodle, Progresso	2
Beef, w/veggies & pasta	2
Clam chowder, red	2
Clam chowder, red, Progresso	2
French onion, no ch, 1 cup	2
Ham and bean	2
Tomato, made w/water	2
Vegetable	2
Vegetable beef	2
Vegetarian beef	2
Won Ton	2
Chicken	3
Chicken broth	3
Chicken gumbo, w/saus	3
Chicken rice, hearty	3
Cream of tomato	3
Lentil	3
Minestrone	3

* Unless otherwise indicated, counts are based on one-cup
servings.

143

SOUP*: Part 2

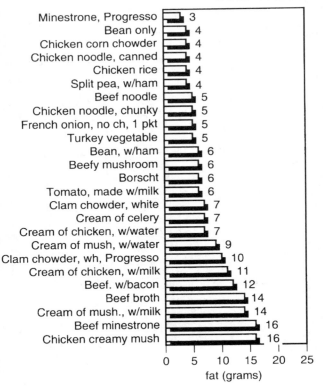

Soup	fat (grams)
Minestrone, Progresso	3
Bean only	4
Chicken corn chowder	4
Chicken noodle, canned	4
Chicken rice	4
Split pea, w/ham	4
Beef noodle	5
Chicken noodle, chunky	5
French onion, no ch, 1 pkt	5
Turkey vegetable	5
Bean, w/ham	6
Beefy mushroom	6
Borscht	6
Tomato, made w/milk	6
Clam chowder, white	7
Cream of celery	7
Cream of chicken, w/water	7
Cream of mush, w/water	9
Clam chowder, wh, Progresso	10
Cream of chicken, w/milk	11
Beef. w/bacon	12
Beef broth	14
Cream of mush., w/milk	14
Beef minestrone	16
Chicken creamy mush	16

fat (grams)

* Unless otherwise indicated, counts are based on one-cup
   servings.

144

Sweets: CAKES*, Part 1

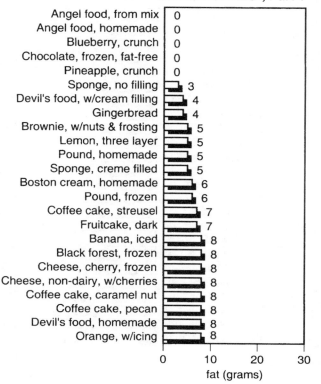

	fat (grams)
Angel food, from mix	0
Angel food, homemade	0
Blueberry, crunch	0
Chocolate, frozen, fat-free	0
Pineapple, crunch	0
Sponge, no filling	3
Devil's food, w/cream filling	4
Gingerbread	4
Brownie, w/nuts & frosting	5
Lemon, three layer	5
Pound, homemade	5
Sponge, creme filled	5
Boston cream, homemade	6
Pound, frozen	6
Coffee cake, streusel	7
Fruitcake, dark	7
Banana, iced	8
Black forest, frozen	8
Cheese, cherry, frozen	8
Cheese, non-dairy, w/cherries	8
Coffee cake, caramel nut	8
Coffee cake, pecan	8
Devil's food, homemade	8
Orange, w/icing	8

* Counts are based on average-size pieces and slices,
  where appropriate, as indicated on package.

Sweets: CAKES*, Part 2

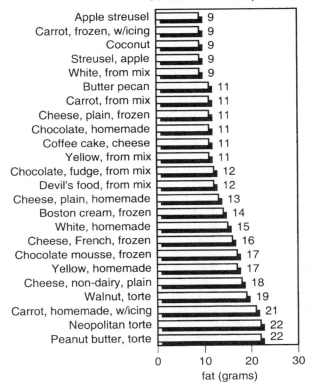

Cake	fat (grams)
Apple streusel	9
Carrot, frozen, w/icing	9
Coconut	9
Streusel, apple	9
White, from mix	9
Butter pecan	11
Carrot, from mix	11
Cheese, plain, frozen	11
Chocolate, homemade	11
Coffee cake, cheese	11
Yellow, from mix	11
Chocolate, fudge, from mix	12
Devil's food, from mix	12
Cheese, plain, homemade	13
Boston cream, frozen	14
White, homemade	15
Cheese, French, frozen	16
Chocolate mousse, frozen	17
Yellow, homemade	17
Cheese, non-dairy, plain	18
Walnut, torte	19
Carrot, homemade, w/icing	21
Neopolitan torte	22
Peanut butter, torte	22

fat (grams): 0 — 10 — 20 — 30

* Counts are based on average-size servings.

146

Sweets: SNACK CAKES*

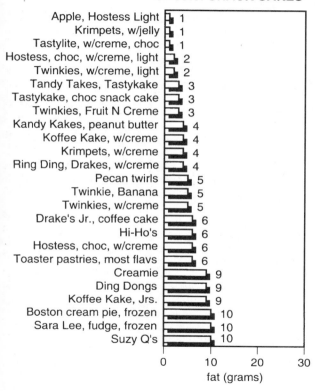

	fat (grams)
Apple, Hostess Light	1
Krimpets, w/jelly	1
Tastylite, w/creme, choc	1
Hostess, choc, w/creme, light	2
Twinkies, w/creme, light	2
Tandy Takes, Tastykake	3
Tastykake, choc snack cake	3
Twinkies, Fruit N Creme	3
Kandy Kakes, peanut butter	4
Koffee Kake, w/creme	4
Krimpets, w/creme	4
Ring Ding, Drakes, w/creme	4
Pecan twirls	5
Twinkie, Banana	5
Twinkies, w/creme	5
Drake's Jr., coffee cake	6
Hi-Ho's	6
Hostess, choc, w/creme	6
Toaster pastries, most flavs	6
Creamie	9
Ding Dongs	9
Koffee Kake, Jrs.	9
Boston cream pie, frozen	10
Sara Lee, fudge, frozen	10
Suzy Q's	10

* Counts are based on average-size pieces and slices,
  where appropriate, as indicated on package.

147

Sweets: CANDY*: Part 1

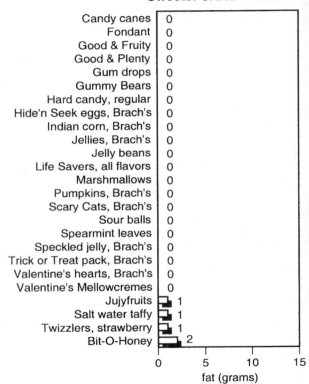

	fat (grams)
Candy canes	0
Fondant	0
Good & Fruity	0
Good & Plenty	0
Gum drops	0
Gummy Bears	0
Hard candy, regular	0
Hide'n Seek eggs, Brach's	0
Indian corn, Brach's	0
Jellies, Brach's	0
Jelly beans	0
Life Savers, all flavors	0
Marshmallows	0
Pumpkins, Brach's	0
Scary Cats, Brach's	0
Sour balls	0
Spearmint leaves	0
Speckled jelly, Brach's	0
Trick or Treat pack, Brach's	0
Valentine's hearts, Brach's	0
Valentine's Mellowcremes	0
Jujyfruits	1
Salt water taffy	1
Twizzlers, strawberry	1
Bit-O-Honey	2

fat (grams)

* For ease of comparison, counts are based on one-ounce
servings. Adjust counts to reflect quantities consumed.

Sweets: CANDY*, Part 2

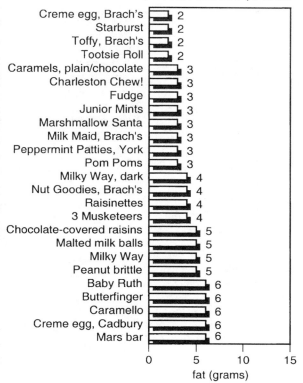

Candy	fat (grams)
Creme egg, Brach's	2
Starburst	2
Toffy, Brach's	2
Tootsie Roll	2
Caramels, plain/chocolate	3
Charleston Chew!	3
Fudge	3
Junior Mints	3
Marshmallow Santa	3
Milk Maid, Brach's	3
Peppermint Patties, York	3
Pom Poms	3
Milky Way, dark	4
Nut Goodies, Brach's	4
Raisinettes	4
3 Musketeers	4
Chocolate-covered raisins	5
Malted milk balls	5
Milky Way	5
Peanut brittle	5
Baby Ruth	6
Butterfinger	6
Caramello	6
Creme egg, Cadbury	6
Mars bar	6

fat (grams)

* For ease of comparison, counts are based on one-ounce
servings. Adjust counts to reflect quantities consumed.

Sweets: CANDY*, Part 3

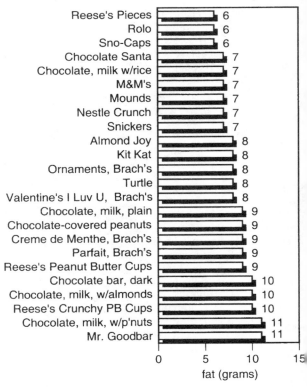

	fat (grams)
Reese's Pieces	6
Rolo	6
Sno-Caps	6
Chocolate Santa	7
Chocolate, milk w/rice	7
M&M's	7
Mounds	7
Nestle Crunch	7
Snickers	7
Almond Joy	8
Kit Kat	8
Ornaments, Brach's	8
Turtle	8
Valentine's I Luv U, Brach's	8
Chocolate, milk, plain	9
Chocolate-covered peanuts	9
Creme de Menthe, Brach's	9
Parfait, Brach's	9
Reese's Peanut Butter Cups	9
Chocolate bar, dark	10
Chocolate, milk, w/almonds	10
Reese's Crunchy PB Cups	10
Chocolate, milk, w/p'nuts	11
Mr. Goodbar	11

* For ease of comparison, counts are based on one-ounce servings. Adjust counts to reflect quantities consumed.

Sweets: COOKIES*, Part 1

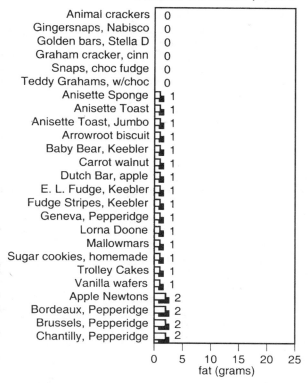

	fat (grams)
Animal crackers	0
Gingersnaps, Nabisco	0
Golden bars, Stella D	0
Graham cracker, cinn	0
Snaps, choc fudge	0
Teddy Grahams, w/choc	0
Anisette Sponge	1
Anisette Toast	1
Anisette Toast, Jumbo	1
Arrowroot biscuit	1
Baby Bear, Keebler	1
Carrot walnut	1
Dutch Bar, apple	1
E. L. Fudge, Keebler	1
Fudge Stripes, Keebler	1
Geneva, Pepperidge	1
Lorna Doone	1
Mallowmars	1
Sugar cookies, homemade	1
Trolley Cakes	1
Vanilla wafers	1
Apple Newtons	2
Bordeaux, Pepperidge	2
Brussels, Pepperidge	2
Chantilly, Pepperidge	2

0   5   10   15   20   25
fat (grams)

* NOTE: For ease of comparison, counts are based on
single cookie servings. When more than one cookie is
consumed, counts should be adjusted accordingly.

Sweets: COOKIES*, Part 2

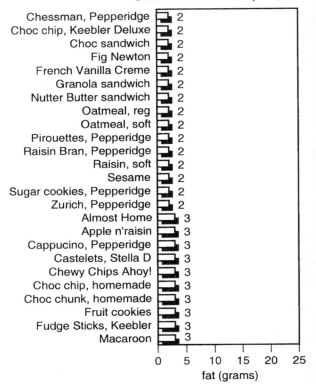

	fat (grams)
Chessman, Pepperidge	2
Choc chip, Keebler Deluxe	2
Choc sandwich	2
Fig Newton	2
French Vanilla Creme	2
Granola sandwich	2
Nutter Butter sandwich	2
Oatmeal, reg	2
Oatmeal, soft	2
Pirouettes, Pepperidge	2
Raisin Bran, Pepperidge	2
Raisin, soft	2
Sesame	2
Sugar cookies, Pepperidge	2
Zurich, Pepperidge	2
Almost Home	3
Apple n'raisin	3
Cappucino, Pepperidge	3
Castelets, Stella D	3
Chewy Chips Ahoy!	3
Choc chip, homemade	3
Choc chunk, homemade	3
Fruit cookies	3
Fudge Sticks, Keebler	3
Macaroon	3

* NOTE: For ease of comparison, counts are based on
single cookie servings. When more than one cookie is
consumed, counts should be adjusted accordingly.

Sweets: COOKIES, Part 3

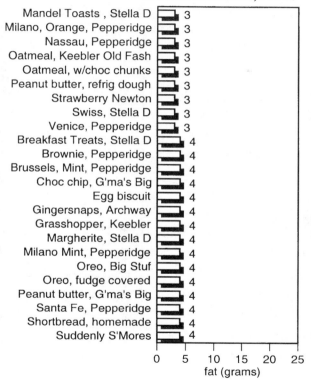

Cookie	fat (grams)
Mandel Toasts , Stella D	3
Milano, Orange, Pepperidge	3
Nassau, Pepperidge	3
Oatmeal, Keebler Old Fash	3
Oatmeal, w/choc chunks	3
Peanut butter, refrig dough	3
Strawberry Newton	3
Swiss, Stella D	3
Venice, Pepperidge	3
Breakfast Treats, Stella D	4
Brownie, Pepperidge	4
Brussels, Mint, Pepperidge	4
Choc chip, G'ma's Big	4
Egg biscuit	4
Gingersnaps, Archway	4
Grasshopper, Keebler	4
Margherite, Stella D	4
Milano Mint, Pepperidge	4
Oreo, Big Stuf	4
Oreo, fudge covered	4
Peanut butter, G'ma's Big	4
Santa Fe, Pepperidge	4
Shortbread, homemade	4
Suddenly S'Mores	4

0   5   10   15   20   25
fat (grams)

* NOTE: For ease of comparison, counts are based on
single cookie servings. When more than one cookie is
consumed, counts should be adjusted accordingly.

Sweets: COOKIES*, Part 4

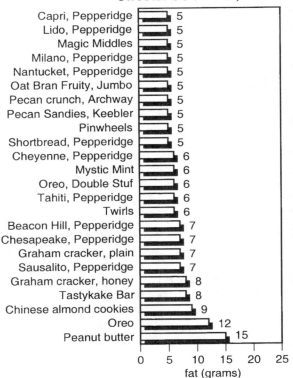

	fat (grams)
Capri, Pepperidge	5
Lido, Pepperidge	5
Magic Middles	5
Milano, Pepperidge	5
Nantucket, Pepperidge	5
Oat Bran Fruity, Jumbo	5
Pecan crunch, Archway	5
Pecan Sandies, Keebler	5
Pinwheels	5
Shortbread, Pepperidge	5
Cheyenne, Pepperidge	6
Mystic Mint	6
Oreo, Double Stuf	6
Tahiti, Pepperidge	6
Twirls	6
Beacon Hill, Pepperidge	7
Chesapeake, Pepperidge	7
Graham cracker, plain	7
Sausalito, Pepperidge	7
Graham cracker, honey	8
Tastykake Bar	8
Chinese almond cookies	9
Oreo	12
Peanut butter	15

* NOTE: For ease of comparison, counts are based on
single cookie servings. When more than one cookie is
consumed, counts should be adjusted accordingly.

Hi-Low Comparison Chart
(for Alphabetical Charts, see pages 1 - 82)

Sweets: DONUTS*

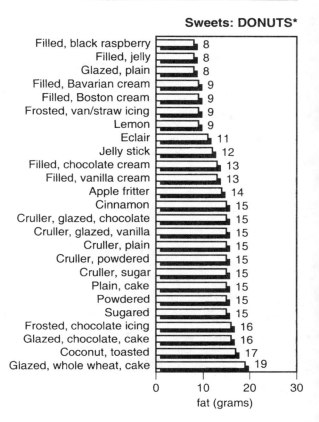

Donut	fat (grams)
Filled, black raspberry	8
Filled, jelly	8
Glazed, plain	8
Filled, Bavarian cream	9
Filled, Boston cream	9
Frosted, van/straw icing	9
Lemon	9
Eclair	11
Jelly stick	12
Filled, chocolate cream	13
Filled, vanilla cream	13
Apple fritter	14
Cinnamon	15
Cruller, glazed, chocolate	15
Cruller, glazed, vanilla	15
Cruller, plain	15
Cruller, powdered	15
Cruller, sugar	15
Plain, cake	15
Powdered	15
Sugared	15
Frosted, chocolate icing	16
Glazed, chocolate, cake	16
Coconut, toasted	17
Glazed, whole wheat, cake	19

* Counts are based on average-size donuts.

155

Sweets: GUM & MINTS*

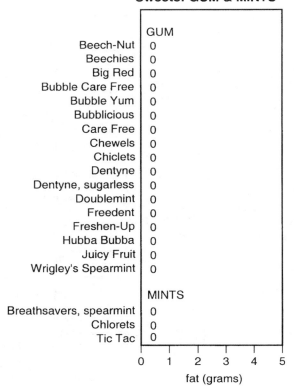

	fat (grams)
GUM	
Beech-Nut	0
Beechies	0
Big Red	0
Bubble Care Free	0
Bubble Yum	0
Bubblicious	0
Care Free	0
Chewels	0
Chiclets	0
Dentyne	0
Dentyne, sugarless	0
Doublemint	0
Freedent	0
Freshen-Up	0
Hubba Bubba	0
Juicy Fruit	0
Wrigley's Spearmint	0
MINTS	
Breathsavers, spearmint	0
Chlorets	0
Tic Tac	0

0   1   2   3   4   5
fat (grams)

* Counts are based on single sticks and mints.

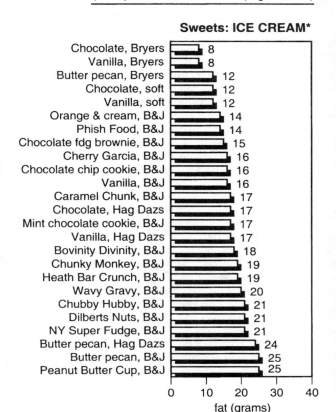

Hi-Low Comparison Chart
(for Alphabetical Charts, see pages 1 - 82)

Sweets: ICE CREAM*

	fat (grams)
Chocolate, Bryers	8
Vanilla, Bryers	8
Butter pecan, Bryers	12
Chocolate, soft	12
Vanilla, soft	12
Orange & cream, B&J	14
Phish Food, B&J	14
Chocolate fdg brownie, B&J	15
Cherry Garcia, B&J	16
Chocolate chip cookie, B&J	16
Vanilla, B&J	16
Caramel Chunk, B&J	17
Chocolate, Hag Dazs	17
Mint chocolate cookie, B&J	17
Vanilla, Hag Dazs	17
Bovinity Divinity, B&J	18
Chunky Monkey, B&J	19
Heath Bar Crunch, B&J	19
Wavy Gravy, B&J	20
Chubby Hubby, B&J	21
Dilberts Nuts, B&J	21
NY Super Fudge, B&J	21
Butter pecan, Hag Dazs	24
Butter pecan, B&J	25
Peanut Butter Cup, B&J	25

0   10   20   30   40
fat (grams)

* Counts are based on one-half cup servings. "B&J"
  designates Ben & Jerry's brand.

157

Sweets: ICE CREAM CONES & BARS, ICE CREAM ALTERNATIVES AND PUDDINGS*

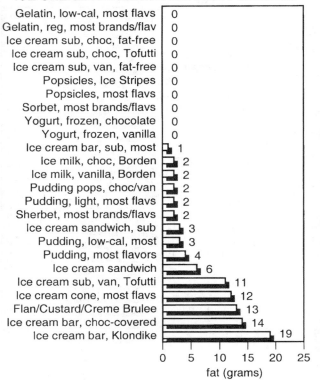

	fat (grams)
Gelatin, low-cal, most flavs	0
Gelatin, reg, most brands/flav	0
Ice cream sub, choc, fat-free	0
Ice cream sub, choc, Tofutti	0
Ice cream sub, van, fat-free	0
Popsicles, Ice Stripes	0
Popsicles, most flavs	0
Sorbet, most brands/flavs	0
Yogurt, frozen, chocolate	0
Yogurt, frozen, vanilla	0
Ice cream bar, sub, most	1
Ice milk, choc, Borden	2
Ice milk, vanilla, Borden	2
Pudding pops, choc/van	2
Pudding, light, most flavs	2
Sherbet, most brands/flavs	2
Ice cream sandwich, sub	3
Pudding, low-cal, most	3
Pudding, most flavors	4
Ice cream sandwich	6
Ice cream sub, van, Tofutti	11
Ice cream cone, most flavs	12
Flan/Custard/Creme Brulee	13
Ice cream bar, choc-covered	14
Ice cream bar, Klondike	19

* Counts are based on average- or one-half cup servings.
  "Sub" designates non-dairy, ice cream substitute.

Sweets: PIES*

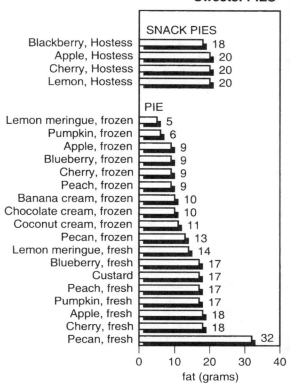

SNACK PIES

Blackberry, Hostess	18
Apple, Hostess	20
Cherry, Hostess	20
Lemon, Hostess	20

PIE

Lemon meringue, frozen	5
Pumpkin, frozen	6
Apple, frozen	9
Blueberry, frozen	9
Cherry, frozen	9
Peach, frozen	9
Banana cream, frozen	10
Chocolate cream, frozen	10
Coconut cream, frozen	11
Pecan, frozen	13
Lemon meringue, fresh	14
Blueberry, fresh	17
Custard	17
Peach, fresh	17
Pumpkin, fresh	17
Apple, fresh	18
Cherry, fresh	18
Pecan, fresh	32

fat (grams)

* Counts are based on average-size pieces and slices,
where appropriate, as indicated on package.

159

Sweets: SUGARS, SYRUPS, TOPPINGS AND JAMS*

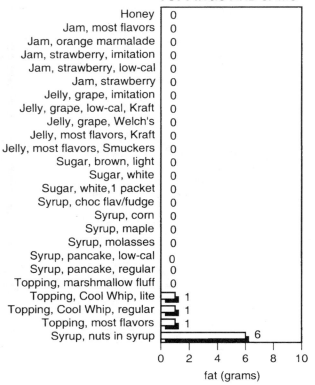

	fat (grams)
Honey	0
Jam, most flavors	0
Jam, orange marmalade	0
Jam, strawberry, imitation	0
Jam, strawberry, low-cal	0
Jam, strawberry	0
Jelly, grape, imitation	0
Jelly, grape, low-cal, Kraft	0
Jelly, grape, Welch's	0
Jelly, most flavors, Kraft	0
Jelly, most flavors, Smuckers	0
Sugar, brown, light	0
Sugar, white	0
Sugar, white, 1 packet	0
Syrup, choc flav/fudge	0
Syrup, corn	0
Syrup, maple	0
Syrup, molasses	0
Syrup, pancake, low-cal	0
Syrup, pancake, regular	0
Topping, marshmallow fluff	0
Topping, Cool Whip, lite	1
Topping, Cool Whip, regular	1
Topping, most flavors	1
Syrup, nuts in syrup	6

* Counts are based on single-tablespoon servings. Jams and preserves can be assumed to have equal values.

160

VEGETABLES*, Part 1

	fat (grams)
Alfalfa sprouts	0
Artichokes, 1 large	0
Asparagus, 6 spears	0
Bean sprouts, mung	0
Beans, green	0
Beets	0
Cabbage, Chinese, cooked	0
Cabbage, green, cooked	0
Cabbage, green, raw	0
Cabbage, red, raw	0
Cabbage, Savoy, raw	0
Carrots, cooked	0
Carrots, raw	0
Cauliflower	0
Celery, 1 stalk	0
Corn, frozen, cooked	0
Cucumber	0
Eggplant	0
Endive	0
Kohlrabi, stems	0
Lettuce, Boston, 1/4 head	0
Lettuce, Cos, 1/4 head	0
Lettuce, Iceberg, 1/4 head	0
Lettuce, Romaine, 1/4 head	0
Mung bean, sprouted	0

```
0    5    10    15    20    25
           fat (grams)
```

* Unless otherwise indicated, counts are based on one-cup servings. For vegetable juices, see the Fruits & Juices section.

VEGETABLES*, Part 2

	fat (grams)
Mushrooms, raw	0
Okra pods, 3 pods	0
Onions , cooked	0
Onions , raw	0
Parsnips	0
Pea pods, Chinese, cooked	0
Peppers, green, raw	0
Peppers, hot chili, 6	0
Peppers, red, raw	0
Plantain, cooked & sliced	0
Potato, baked, 1 medium	0
Potato, sweet	0
Radishes, raw, 5 large	0
Sauerkraut	0
Seaweed, kelp, raw	0
Spinach, cooked	0
Spinach, raw	0
Tomato puree	0
Tomato sauce	0
Turnip greens	0
Turnips, cooked	0
Water chestnuts, canned	0
Bamboo shoots	1
Broccoli, 1 spear	1
Brussels sprouts	1

0   5   10   15   20   25

fat (grams)

* Unless otherwise indicated, counts are based on one-cup
servings. For vegetable juices, see the Fruits & Juices
section.

VEGETABLES*, Part 3

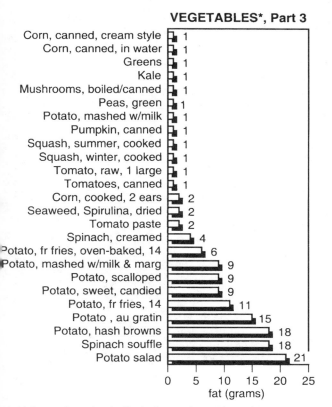

	fat (grams)
Corn, canned, cream style	1
Corn, canned, in water	1
Greens	1
Kale	1
Mushrooms, boiled/canned	1
Peas, green	1
Potato, mashed w/milk	1
Pumpkin, canned	1
Squash, summer, cooked	1
Squash, winter, cooked	1
Tomato, raw, 1 large	1
Tomatoes, canned	1
Corn, cooked, 2 ears	2
Seaweed, Spirulina, dried	2
Tomato paste	2
Spinach, creamed	4
Potato, fr fries, oven-baked, 14	6
Potato, mashed w/milk & marg	9
Potato, scalloped	9
Potato, sweet, candied	9
Potato, fr fries, 14	11
Potato , au gratin	15
Potato, hash browns	18
Spinach souffle	18
Potato salad	21

0   5   10   15   20   25
fat (grams)

* Unless otherwise indicated, counts are based on one-cup
servings. For vegetable juices, see the Fruits & Juices
section.

163

VEGETARIAN CHOICES*

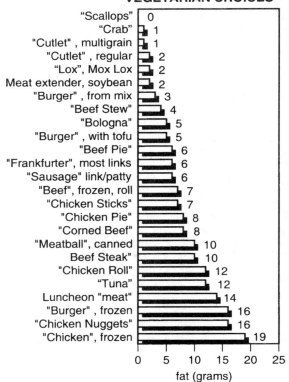

Item	fat (grams)
"Scallops"	0
"Crab"	1
"Cutlet", multigrain	1
"Cutlet", regular	2
"Lox", Mox Lox	2
Meat extender, soybean	2
"Burger", from mix	3
"Beef Stew"	4
"Bologna"	5
"Burger", with tofu	5
"Beef Pie"	6
"Frankfurter", most links	6
"Sausage" link/patty	6
"Beef", frozen, roll	7
"Chicken Sticks"	7
"Chicken Pie"	8
"Corned Beef"	8
"Meatball", canned	10
Beef Steak"	10
"Chicken Roll"	12
"Tuna"	12
Luncheon "meat"	14
"Burger", frozen	16
"Chicken Nuggets"	16
"Chicken", frozen	19

fat (grams)

* Made from tofu, textured vegetable protein or a combination of both. Counts are based on 3-ounce servings.

PLUME

From Drs. Richard F. and Rachael F. Heller

THE CARBOHYDRATE ADDICT'S LIFESPAN PROGRAM
The phenomenal weight-loss program that teaches you how to break your addiction to carbohydrates while enjoying food as you never have before.

0-452-27838-4

**THE CARBOHYDRATE ADDICT'S PROGRAM
FOR SUCCESS**
The companion workbook to *The Carbohydrate Addict's LifeSpan Program*, this essential volume provides additional tools, resources, and support for carbohydrate addicts using this breakthrough program.

0-452-26933-4

HEALTHY FOR LIFE
Reduce your risk of heart disease, diabetes, stroke, cancer, and high blood pressure—without deprivation or sacrifice—through this revolutionary nutritional program designed for lifetime success.

0-452-27112-6